Testimonials from some of the several thousand people who have already benefited from the Metabolism Miracle program:

"The Metabolism Miracle program has helped me to deflate the spare tire around my middle. But this plan is about more than just weight loss. It is a lifestyle change that has improved my self-confidence and energy level along with my waistline."
—*Leighe Weifert*

"I've spent much of my adult life trying to diet, count calories, and curtail sweets. I've lost and gained weight many times over. My blood sugar levels were beginning to rise, and I was concerned about diabetes. Diane's program has been the one that enabled me to lose weight and inches, to eat regular foods, and to maintain my goal weight over time. My blood sugar has returned to normal, and I am no longer prediabetic. The Metabolism Miracle program works!"—*Bonnie Rynar, DMD*

"When I first started Step One, I was twenty years old, 278 pounds, and extremely unhappy. I had already seen a gastroenterologist about having gastric bypass surgery and felt that was my only option. I had no hope left. My family convinced me to try this diet first, and it changed my life. Two months into Step One and I had lost 21 pounds. It was easy, life changing, and, best of all, no surgery was involved!"—*Melissa Ricca*

"Diane Kress literally saved my life with the Metabolism Miracle. When I first met Diane, my sugar levels were completely out of control. I was 50 pounds overweight, and my energy level was practically nonexistent. I was desperate and I knew if I didn't change my lifestyle my diabetes would do me in. In my eyes Diane Kress is a miracle worker. Step One, with its boot camp/rehab/detox, was a major diet change. And in Step Two—transition and retraining—I started to see progress. My energy levels got better, and my lab work improved significantly. In eight months I went from 230 pounds to 186 pounds. I will be indebted to Diane Kress forever. I'm truly a believer." —JL

"This diet really has been a metabolism miracle for me. During Step One, I could feel my energy rise as my cravings disappeared and I lost pounds and inches. On Step Two, as I retrained my body to process carbohydrates properly, I found myself reassessing my relationship with food and the role my moods play in my eating habits. I am now a more conscious eater and take better care of my emotional as well as physical self. I will stay on Step Two until I am truly centered. I look forward to the next stage of my life, with Step Three playing a vital role. The Metabolism Miracle is a welcome, integral part of my life." —A grateful patient

"This program has brought a marked change to my life. Not only have I reduced my body fat, but my energy level, mood, and focus have skyrocketed. Coming from a long line of family members with type 2 diabetes and high cholesterol, committing to this program has given me the control to prevent these previously eventual endpoints. It is truly remarkable." —Elana Walker

"The Metabolism Miracle deserves to stand out from the crowd. The great ease of the lifestyle program is something I am truly excited about. I even made it through all the holidays without having to cheat! I struggled for years trying to lose weight and all I seemed to do was gain. With the help of this program I have lost 42 pounds, and I have improved energy levels. I can finally say that I have my life back!" —Tara Grande

"I am a sixty-six-year-old woman. Up until the age of fifty-two, I was an absolute vision to behold! It was downhill from there. On the recommendation of my endocrinologist, I went to see Diane

Kress. I was unaware that there was a reason for my lack of energy and weight gain. I was the poster girl for the metabolic syndrome, with high blood pressure, prediabetic numbers, thyroid instability, and high cholesterol. This diet has allowed me to get my groove back! After my trying and failing all other diets, the Metabolism Miracle was miraculous for me! My before and after blood work is proudly displayed in a frame on my wall."—*DO*

"Not only has the Metabolism Miracle enabled me to make positive lifestyle changes for the present, but it will also prove to be the lifesaving program that I will follow for the rest of my life."
—*Scott Seiferheld*

"In 2001 I had a heart attack and underwent bypass surgery that was complicated by diabetes. I then turned to Diane Kress, who with persuasion, humor, and discipline taught me a new lifestyle program. It was simple and succeeded in helping me thrive and enjoy life without too much anxiety."—*A patient*

"I am absolutely thrilled with the results I obtained following Diane Kress's Metabolism Miracle program. I lost over 20 pounds and more significantly, 8 inches in my waist. Moreover, I did not lose muscle mass, which is very important to me as a fit and active senior."—*Jerry Glick*

"The Metabolism Miracle program changed my life in so many good ways. I am medication and insulin-free, have more energy, and at sixty-seven years, feel like I am in my forties—and credit all to your program. Thank you for giving me a better way to eat and control my diabetes. You enhanced my life and I am forever grateful to you."—*Arnold Schancupp, Esq.*

THE
METABOLISM
MIRACLE

3 Easy Steps to Regain
Control of Your Weight . . . Permanently

DIANE KRESS, RD, CDE

Da Capo
LIFE
LONG

A MEMBER OF THE PERSEUS BOOKS GROUP

Set in 11 point Electra by the Perseus Books Group

Cataloging-in-Publication data for this book is available from the Library of Congress.

HC ISBN: 978-0-7382-1277-7
PB ISBN: 978-0-7382-1386-6
First Da Capo Press edition 2009
First Da Capo Press paperback edition 2010

Note: The information in this book is true and complete to the best of our knowledge. This book is intended only as an informative guide for those wishing to know more about health issues. In no way is this book intended to replace, countermand, or conflict with the advice given to you by your own physician. The ultimate decision concerning care should be made between you and your doctor. We strongly recommend you follow his or her advice. Information in this book is general and is offered with no guarantees on the part of the authors of Da Capo Press. The authors and publisher disclaim all liability in connection with the use of this book. The names and identifying details of people associated with events described in this book have been changed. Any similarity to actual persons is coincidental.

Published by Da Capo Press
A Member of the Perseus Books Group
www.dacapopress.com

Da Capo Press books are available at special discounts for bulk purchases in the United States by corporations, institutions, and other organizations. For more information, please contact the Special Markets Department at the Perseus Books Group, 2300 Chestnut Street, Suite 200, Philadelphia, PA 19103, or call (800) 255-1514, or e-mail special.markets@perseusbooks.com.

6 7 8 9 10

THIS BOOK IS DEDICATED WITH LOVE AND GRATITUDE TO

JC and Therese

Contents

PART THREE

Exploring Health and Life Issues

PART FOUR

Recipes

Introduction

A Plan for Your Body

In over twenty-five years, working with thousands of patients, I've met countless frustrated dieters. They walk through my office door, sit down across the desk from me, and describe their unsuccessful efforts to lose weight and keep it off. They often tell me that my office will be their last stop: "If this program doesn't work, I am giving up."

Diet after diet, pounds lost, pounds regained, they keep trying, they keep hoping, and yet they never get lasting results.

That all changes when they walk through my office door. By choosing this book, you've walked through the same door.

Diets are built on the assumption that everyone's metabolism works in the same way and that the diet that works for one person will work equally well for another. In other words, metabolism is metabolism and one size fits all. But what if your metabolism doesn't quite match the textbook version? What if your body works a little differently than the standard? What if you weren't failing at dieting, but your diet was failing you?

In fact, over 50 percent of patients seen in my practice for weight loss and weight-related health issues, as well as millions of people across the country and worldwide, really do have a very different metabolism than the type described as "normal." These people have tried diet after diet, having faithfully followed the rules that have produced results for their friends. Unbeknownst to them, those weight-loss programs can never work because they don't match the metabolism of these individuals.

If you find it impossible to lose weight and keep it off, even when you follow all the rules, there's an excellent chance that your metabolism doesn't match the cookie-cutter kind. The Metabolism Miracle was designed for people like you, to help you understand your body and learn to work with it rather than against it.

The Metabolism Miracle is not just another diet book. The program is the result of twenty-five years of working with thousands of patients whose metabolism did not follow the expected norm. Before I discovered the way to fuel this metabolism properly, they had little to no chance of permanent weight loss, no matter how hard they tried. Now they walk out my door with the potential for 100 percent success.

BE PREPARED TO BE SURPRISED

On any given day, over 35 percent of Americans—more than 71 million people—actively try to lose weight. As a result, the weight-loss industry has exploded with gimmicks and fads all promising a "slimmer, sexier, healthier you."

Yet as you look around, you will see more overweight people than ever before. More than 60 percent of the population is classified as overweight and the numbers are escalating. Americans spend billions of dollars annually in the pursuit of quick, easy, and lasting weight loss. Ironically, as we spend more time, energy, and money than ever to lose weight, our population is heavier than ever before.

We are becoming sicker as a consequence. Many serious conditions are linked directly to weight. The risks of type 2 diabetes, cardiovascular disease, cancer, hypertension, acid reflux disease, sleep apnea, depression, and even infertility all increase as weight increases.

The long-term success rate of any of the available diet plans is a meager 2 percent. That means only two out of one hundred serious dieters have been able to maintain their weight loss at the end of five years. Ninety percent of dieters who have managed to lose weight regain all of it within one year! As a result, people jump from diet to diet, hoping to find the magic formula that will help them to lose unhealthy weight and keep it off for a lifetime. They spend years of their lives counting calories, spending "points," weighing and measuring food as well as their bodies, checking fat grams, checking sugar grams, and ultimately punishing themselves for falling off their program.

The Metabolism Miracle breaks through this dieting madness. For years, medical science recognized a one-size-fits-all metabolism and standard diet programs were designed accordingly. More recently, researchers identified an alternative metabolism and categorized it under a variety of terms, including *metabolic syndrome, syndrome* X, and *insulin resistance*. Millions of people have this alternative metabolism, which I refer to as *Metabolism B*. Unfortunately a diet has never been fully developed to work in tandem with all the special requirements of this type of metabolism. Up until now, there was no diet to rely upon for permanent weight loss.

If you have Metabolism B, you were born with a different blueprint for processing food. You may not always have had problems keeping weight off, but at some point over the years the progressive nature of Metabolism B advanced to the point that you noticed the symptoms: progressive weight gain around the middle, fatigue, and carb cravings. Unchecked, the symptoms lead to health issues involving cholesterol, blood sugar, and blood pressure. Your body no longer abides by the dieting rules that work for others. Instead, you require a program that has been designed with your blueprint in mind.

The Metabolism Miracle program is a three-step approach that resists your body's overactive response to carbohydrate, trains your body to handle carbohydrate normally, and then teaches you to live a life in harmony with your unique metabolism. Once you learn to live in balance with your metabolism, your weight will come off and *permanently* stay off. Your health will improve, your energy level will soar, and you'll experience a feeling of peace and contentment. Miraculously, you will begin to feel the effects of this new approach in less than one week.

To determine if you have Metabolism B, you will complete a basic checklist that pinpoints the telltale signs, symptoms, and personal medical history that characterize people with Metabolism B. If you would like more in-depth proof, your most recent lab data can verify the results. Either way, your search for the right weight-loss program has ended.

The Metabolism Miracle will help you to understand the way your body works and empower you to work with your metabolism instead of against it. The Miracle will bring back the healthy you—no more carb cravings, energy slumps, food binges, or frustrating weight regain. You will learn about the foods that you can eat whenever you are hungry, with no calorie counting, weighing, or measuring. You'll also learn about the energy foods that will fuel your metabolism all day long. Weight-related health problems will diminish and even disappear. And you will feel healthier and more energized than you have felt in years or perhaps in your lifetime.

The Metabolism Miracle is easy, effective, and, best of all, the first and only program written expressly for *you*.

PART ONE

Your Metabolism Is Different

A PROGRAM TO CHANGE YOUR LIFE

You know who you are.

You have suffered through liquid diets, portion-controlled diets, calorie-counting diets, point diets, fat-free diets, carb-free diets, grapefruit diets, and doctor diets, only to regain every pound you lost. You sit at weight-loss support meetings next to people who succeed while you do not. You are an expert in dieting. You can recite the calorie content of foods without glancing at a book. You have tried, over and over. *You really have tried.*

Yet you have known for a long time that something is very different about your body. Others eat twice the quantity of food that you consume, and they weigh much less than you. No matter what the doctors and nutritionists say, you insist that you must have a different metabolism.

You are right.

I know this, because, like you, I have this different metabolism and it confounded me for much of my life. *The Metabolism Miracle* is the culmination of my life's work in treating people with stubborn weight and weight-related maladies. But the story began with my own body. I have spent more than twenty-five years as a registered dietitian specializing in weight loss, prevention and management of diabetes, and cardiovascular nutrition. Only after my own health declined and I pieced together clues from years of personal trial and error, the experience of thousands of patients, and current medical research, did I finally find the answer.

The Metabolism Miracle changed my life and continues to keep my patients and me healthier than ever before.

A PERSONAL STORY

As a registered dietitian, trained in the traditional approach to nutrition, I have counseled thousands of people over the years and worked equally hard with all of them. Yet early in my clinical practice, I noticed something that deeply concerned me. More than 45 percent of those I counseled never achieved their desired results.

In the traditional school of thought, a person will gain weight if he or she consumes more calories than are burned off. Most weight loss diets are based on this "law of calories." The fewer calories a person consumes, the less he or she will weigh. Add physical activity to the equation and weight loss accelerates. But the law of calories didn't apply to all of my patients.

For years, I used a universal formula for all of my weight-loss clients to determine the number of calories they should consume to lose weight. I dutifully plugged my patients' gender, height, desired weight, age, and physical activity into the formula and came up with a calorie allotment that should have guaranteed their weight loss. If the patient's cholesterol was elevated, I added a saturated fat and dietary cholesterol restriction. If they suffered from hypertension, I added a sodium restriction. The formula then configured a nice, neat diet package with precise calorie allotments.

The patients followed the diet, weighed and measured food portions, kept detailed food journals, and exercised regularly. But many of them returned for their follow-up visit disillusioned and depressed.

Nothing significant had happened! They had lost little weight and had no real change in their blood lipids, blood sugar, or blood pressure. They remained on medications and, worse yet, their medications increased over the years.

I sympathized, but I also wondered if they had truly followed my instructions. Perhaps they wrote what they believed I wanted to see in their food logs. Maybe, in reality, they didn't follow the plan or exercise. Perhaps they were overeating or sneaking in snacks. The diet worked for half of my clients, so why didn't it work for all of them?

As time passed, I realized that if I were to help these patients, I would have to challenge some of the principles that were written in stone by the medical community. There had to be a reason for the obesity epidemic. Why was type 2 diabetes afflicting more and younger people? Why were so few people succeeding at diets despite the billion-dollar weight-loss industry? Why were we becoming a nation reliant on prescription medications? Something had to be very wrong with the theories.

Then something alarming happened to me.

As a nutrition counselor with a thriving practice, I knew everything there was to know about diets; I could configure them in my sleep. I prided myself in following a balanced, healthful diet. I exercised regularly and practiced what I preached. But as I entered my thirties, my body changed.

At a routine physical exam, a nurse told me that my consistently low blood pressure had increased to the normal zone. Shortly after, my cholesterol and triglyceride levels began to rise, regardless of exercise and a low-fat, low-cholesterol lifestyle. Soon, even as I counted every calorie that passed my lips, the numbers on the scale began to creep upward. Worse yet, I noticed a small roll of fat around my middle!

I followed the guidelines that I had been taught were the key to good health. Like my patients, I monitored my calories, fat, cholesterol, and sodium, and I exercised faithfully. Despite all of this effort, I continued to gain weight and eventually needed medication to help control my blood pressure and cholesterol.

Finally, just before my fortieth birthday, I developed type 2 diabetes. What had happened? Nothing I did would stop this train! Despite my attempts to do everything by the book, my body would not respond. I finally felt the full force of the frustration and emotional pain that my patients endured.

The experience led me right back to the traditional nutrition theories that I had been teaching my patients. This time, I dug into the research, analyzed the nutrition "wisdom," and looked at the patterns that fit my successful patients and unsuccessful patients. I tested out new approaches, threw out those that didn't work, and came up with confirmation of what I had come to suspect: It was clear that one segment of dieters responded to the traditional approach. The other needed a very different and new approach. The Metabolism Miracle is that approach.

It worked. Within the first few weeks on the program, I felt like a new person, with higher energy, looser jeans, and no cravings. Within the second month, my doctor eliminated my hypertension medication and decreased my medication for cholesterol. Eventually, I no longer needed any of my medications and my blood pressure, cholesterol, weight, and diabetes remained under good control! I felt great and friends told me I looked ten years younger.

Not only did the program work for me, it worked for each patient who followed it. I erased the board of all the ideals I had once held as dietary gospel and I rewrote the diet book.

A DIFFERENT KIND OF METABOLISM

Most weight-loss advice recognizes only one metabolism, the version every medical student and dietetics student is currently taught. I call this *Metabolism* A. But as I failed to lose weight on standard diets written for Metabolism A, and as I watched many of my patients fail to lose weight on those diets, it became clear that we were working with a different animal, a metabolism that I refer to as *Metabolism B*. This alternative metabolism requires an entirely different approach and that is how the Metabolism Miracle began to take shape.

You may be familiar with the labels *metabolic syndrome* and *insulin resistance*, terms designed by the medical community to recognize alternative metabolism. Together with a host of other signs that may seem unrelated, including fatigue, sleeplessness, mild depression, and anxiety, these conditions point to Metabolism B. Although alternative metabolism has been recognized for years, no diet to date addresses all the facets that contribute to this metabolism. As a result, all diets designed to match alternative metabolism have fallen short. The Metabolism Miracle takes the whole package of symptoms into account, stops the weight-gain train in its tracks, and even helps to reverse some of the health consequences of this metabolism.

Individuals with Metabolism B will never succeed at following a traditional weight-loss diet because their alternative metabolism follows a different set of rules than those of the standard metabolism. In fact, attempting to lose weight using a traditional approach can set off the downward spiral of unchecked Metabolism B.

The split between dieters with Metabolism A and Metabolism B is almost even. More than 45 percent of those struggling to lose weight were born with the genetic predisposition to Metabolism B. The onset of their symptoms is slow and progressive and may be expedited by a number of life events, including stress, weight gain, illness, and hormonal changes.

Take heart. You do not lack willpower! You are not a lazy dieter! You have not imagined impossible obstacles! Your body simply responds differently. Once you understand your body, you can work with your unique metabolism instead of against it. By identifying the category you were born into, you can easily make the right food choices to lead a healthy life at your healthy weight.

Because other diets haven't worked for people with Metabolism B, permanent weight loss can feel overwhelmingly difficult and often downright impossible. Add a health issue such as type 2 diabetes to the scenario and the extra weight becomes downright scary. I know because I've been there.

If you have the genes that have set you up for a lifetime of struggles with weight, The Metabolism Miracle will absolutely work for you. Before the Metabolism Miracle, you had little to no chance of permanent weight loss. With the program, you will reach and maintain a healthy weight, your lab data will improve, the dose of medications that you take to control weight-related health problems will decrease or disappear and you may avoid health risks down the line.

Best of all, you will look and feel great!

IS THIS YOU?

Anyone can lose weight with *The Metabolism Miracle*, but the program is designed specifically for people who have Metabolism B and therefore have no chance of long-term weight loss success with any other diet plan. They will, for the first time, lose weight and *successfully* keep it off for the rest of their lives because this approach, unlike other weight-loss programs, matches their unique metabolism.

You may be saying, "I must not have Metabolism B because only two years ago I could control my weight with no problem." Keep in mind that people with Metabolism B have always had the genetic predisposition for this alternative metabolism but it is only when an outside trigger, such as stress, weight, inactivity, or illness, flips the switch that Metabolism B begins to manifest itself in such symptoms as weight gain or high cholesterol. Some people show symptoms as children and others show symptoms during the teen or adult years. The longer a person has been living with unchecked Metabolism B in its switched-on mode, the more progressive their weight gain and weight-related health issues become. *(See "Trouble Triggers," page 30.)*

How do you know if you have this alternate metabolism? When a patient walks into my office, often on a referral from a medical doctor, I listen to their weight-loss history and get a sense of their overall

9

health, energy, and well-being. I review their family medical history, and if they have a blood profile from a recent visit to the doctor, I screen those numbers. All of these clues help me to identify whether the patient has Metabolism A or B. This chapter will help you to do the same.

To start, answer the following twelve descriptive questions. Most people with Metabolism B see themselves as they answer "yes" to questions on the list. If you recognize yourself in a number of them, you may have Metabolism B and you should move on to the easy checklists that follow.

A LOOK IN THE MIRROR

_____ Have you dieted for years, perhaps successfully in the past, but now even tried-and-true diets you once relied upon for weight loss fail you?

_____ Do you notice that you can only stick to a diet for a short time and you get so discouraged by the dismal results, constant hunger, and overwhelming cravings that you abandon your good intentions?

_____ Are you gaining weight regardless of your efforts and is this weight shifting into a roll around your middle?

_____ Does the fat around your midsection look and feel spongy, loose, and watery?

_____ Can people around you can eat more and yet weigh less than you?

_____ Is your overall health—physical, mental, and emotional— declining as your weight increases?

_____ Do you need medical prescriptions for weight-related health problems such as hypertension, cholesterol, triglycerides, acid reflux, insomnia, depression, anxiety, or arthritis pain?

_____ Despite diet and exercise, has your doctor been forced to increase your medication dosages or add new prescriptions to maintain your health?

_____ Do cravings sometimes gnaw at you like an addiction and do you feel a strong urge to eat carbohydrates such as candy, sweets, bread, pasta, or chips?

_____ Do you feel depressed, irritable, unattractive, and undesirable?

_____ Are you fatigued, even after a proper amount of sleep?

_____ Do you miss the "old you"?

If you found yourself answering yes to several of these questions, go directly to the following simple checklist of symptoms to learn whether the Metabolism Miracle can help you regain your health and sense of well-being and lose weight forever. If you answer no to all of these checkpoints, it's quite possible that you have textbook metabolism, Metabolism A, and can lose weight on any good weight-loss program.

CLUES TO METABOLISM B

This list of symptoms is one of the first pieces of information I use when trying to identify Metabolism A or Metabolism B. It still surprises me that when people with Metabolism A read the checklist, they only identify with a few of the symptoms, whereas people with Metabolism B relate to many, if not most of them.

Check off any of the following experiences that describe a day in your life.

_____ You tire easily and frequently feel fatigued, even upon awakening.

_____ You feel mildly depressed.

_____ You feel an energy slump in the late afternoon.

_____ You frequently feel anxious.

_____ You crave carbohydrate foods, such as bread, chips, sweets, or pasta.

_____ Your midsection has a roll of fat.

_____ You gain weight easily and find it difficult to lose weight.

_____ You have trouble sleeping.

_____ You are often forgetful and worry about your short-term memory.

_____ You have racing thoughts.

_____ Your sexual drive has declined.

_____ You find it difficult to focus and concentrate and are easily distracted.

_____ Bright light or headlights at night bother you.

_____ You are irritable and have a "short fuse."

_____ You have increased sensitivity to aches and pains.

_____ Your eyes frequently tear up and at other times feel dry and irritated.

_____ You have frequent dull headaches.

_____ You feel slightly dizzy, flushed, or "weak in the knees" after even a little bit of alcohol.

If you have identified with twelve or more of the clues on this symptoms checklist, you likely have Metabolism B.

You may have looked at the symptoms checklist for Metabolism B and thought that they could be attributed to many different conditions, including menopause, chronic fatigue syndrome, midlife, or even a high-stress job. But at the end of eight weeks on Step One of the Metabolism Miracle, many symptoms from the checklist will disappear along with weight because the symptoms stem from untreated Metabolism B.

Any symptoms that persist are related to something else and should be addressed from another angle. For example, if after eight weeks a patient still has panic attacks, it would be prudent to discuss them with his or her physician.

ANN'S EPIPHANY

When Ann first came to my Nutrition Center she checked off many of the symptoms from the checklist. She smiled when she handed the list to me, saying, "Of course, I feel this way. These symptoms are due to menopause and, honey, I'm there."

I agreed that the symptoms could relate to many conditions—menopause, fibromyalgia, chronic fatigue syndrome, and just plain aging. But once people begin the Metabolism Miracle program, they quickly discover whether their metabolism may be to blame for many of the unpleasant symptoms.

Ann started the three-step Metabolism Miracle program and, a few weeks later, she sent me an e-mail message with only two words: "It lifted." When she returned to the office after eight weeks, she was beaming. "I can't believe it! Almost all of the symptoms I attributed to menopause—my mild depression, periods of anxiety, poor sleep, midline fat, weight gain, fatigue, forgetfulness—are all so much better." Ann had lost inches of fat and was already wearing smaller-size slacks, but mostly she was thrilled to feel like her old self again.

Still, she couldn't understand why one symptom hadn't changed. "I am still irritable and have a short fuse."

I had to laugh and explain that the program can't fix everything. "Ann, you are just plain irritable with a short fuse!"

BLAME IT ON THE GENES: 22 HEALTH CONDITIONS AFFECTED BY METABOLISM B

Certain medical conditions are very common in people with Metabolism B. They range from high cholesterol to type 2 diabetes. The longer you live your life without treating Metabolism B properly, the greater the chance that you will develop some of these medical problems. The sooner you start the Metabolism Miracle, the more likely you are to avoid these problems in the future or, as is often the case, the more likely you can reverse them.

Many of these conditions work in a domino-like chain effect, with the genetic profile for Metabolism B starting the reaction. For example, it is Metabolism B's excessive insulin release that causes midline fat to accumulate. That midline fat in turn provokes hypertension and acid reflux (GERD). In another chain, excess insulin in the bloodstream promotes excess circulating fats such as cholesterol and triglycerides, and they in turn contribute to heart disease. Fluctuating blood sugar levels, a direct result of unchecked Metabolism B, can contribute to mild depression, anxiety, panic attacks, and short-term memory loss. Hormonal imbalance can cause polycystic ovarian syndrome and irregularity in menstrual cycles and may even contribute to infertility. You get the picture.

If you are young and haven't experienced any of these conditions, don't wave them off. Look at your family's medical history and ascertain if parents, siblings, grandparents, aunts, or uncles have had any of the following medical conditions.

Almost all of the medical conditions listed below require medication. When you fuel your metabolism correctly, with a measured carbohydrate dose in the strategically timed pattern designed in the Metabolism Miracle, the need for that medication may actually decline. You'll need less medication as you enjoy improved mental, physical, and emotional health, increased energy, and weight loss.

If you've experienced any of the following twenty-two medical conditions, you may want to read more about them and how they relate to your Metabolism B. For a detailed explanation of the following medical conditions, see the glossary.

22 HEALTH CONDITIONS THAT ARE AFFECTED BY METABOLISM B

_____ ADD or ADHD (attention deficit syndrome)
_____ Anxiety or panic attacks

_____ Cholesterol increases: total cholesterol, LDL "bad" cholesterol, and/or triglycerides

_____ Low levels of HDL "good" cholesterol

_____ Chronic fatigue

_____ Mild depression

_____ Prediabetes

_____ Type 2 diabetes

_____ Gestational diabetes (occurs only during pregnancy)

_____ Fibromyalgia

_____ GERD (gastric reflux disease)

_____ High blood pressure or recent increases in blood pressure

_____ Hypoglycemia (low blood sugar)

_____ Hypothyroidism (underactive thyroid—are you taking Synthroid or Levoxyl?)

_____ Infertility related to hormonal imbalance

_____ Metabolic syndrome

_____ Midline fat deposits (a roll around your middle) and increasing weight without increasing food intake

_____ Osteoarthritis

_____ Osteoporosis or osteopenia

_____ PCOS (polycystic ovarian syndrome). Symptoms may include irregular menstrual period, heavy blood flow, clotting, severe PMS, and irregular endocrine reproductive hormonal patterns

_____ Sleep apnea

_____ Sleep disturbances

If you have identified with twelve or more of the clues on the symptoms checklist on page 11, you likely have Metabolism B. If, in addition, you or a close relative currently has or has had several of the twenty-two medical conditions linked to Metabolism B, the case is even stronger for Metabolism B. Still skeptical? You may want to look at your most recent blood profile.

A PEEK AT YOUR NUMBERS

It is not necessary to have lab work done before beginning the Metabolism Miracle program. But if you have had blood work drawn within the past six months, compare your numbers to the Metabolism Miracle target range below. Keep in mind that the ranges used for this program are stricter than the American Medical Association's current recommendations because, not only does the Miracle help you to keep off weight, it also focuses on preventing medical problems in the future.

If you take medication to help control blood pressure, cholesterol, or blood sugar, your findings may appear in the normal range because they are being "Band-Aided." Ask yourself, "If I were not on medication, would these readings be normal?" Remember that this lab work needs to be drawn as *fasting* blood work (taken after at least eight hours without food or calorie-containing beverages).

Place a check on any line in which your numbers fall within the Metabolism B range.

		NORMAL	METABOLISM B
____	*Fasting* blood glucose	65–99	90 or above
____	Total cholesterol	less than 200	200 or above
____	LDL Cholesterol	less than 100	100 or above
____	HDL Cholesterol	greater than 45	less than 45
____	Cholesterol/HDL ratio	less than 5	greater than 4
____	Triglycerides	less than 150	100 or above
____	Hemoglobin A1C	less than 6.0	greater than 6.0
____	Blood pressure	less than 130/80	greater than 130/80

If you checked off a fasting glucose of 90 or above, you have Metabolism B and can rest assured that the Metabolism Miracle will work for you. The more lab results that are out of range, the more influence

Metabolism B has had on your health to this point. One of the goals of the Miracle is to get your lab work as close to normal as possible with as little medication as possible. In as little as eight weeks, your physician may need to lower your dosage of medication as your body enters a healthier zone.

For more information and background on how Metabolism B can lead to blood sugar conditions, please see chapter 12.

FINDING THE HIDDEN HEALTH CLUES

Before attempting any weight-loss program with my patients I must first determine if they have Metabolism A or Metabolism B. Without this clarification, close to half of all dieters will not be able to lose weight permanently because most weight-loss programs do not match their alternative metabolism.

Each clue helps me to build the case for Metabolism B. But it's the whole picture that really tells the story.

JOANNE: A MIDLIFE CRISIS?

Consider the case of forty-three-year-old Joanne who is battling the midlife bulge. A mother of three children who range in age from five to sixteen, Joanne works part-time from her home office, exercises to stay physically fit, and vows to grow older "kicking and screaming."

She called my office in a panic. She explained that she can count calories in her sleep and can recite word for word the mantra of most diet programs. In the past, when her jeans felt snug, Joanne would join a popular diet program along with friends, all of whom seem to be battling weight at some level, and she was able to take off the excess weight in a reasonable amount of time.

Recently, things had changed for reasons that perplexed Joanne. She had been feeling mildly depressed and fatigued and, despite repeated attempts at weight loss, despite increasing her gym visits from three to five days per week, despite using the same diet program that she had always used to lose weight, she could not keep off the pounds. She had developed an annoying paunch and no abdominal workout could budge it.

A self-confessed "carboholic," Joanne said that she was very strict with her eating and aggressive with her workouts. A doctor had once told her she had hypoglycemia but she took no medication and she couldn't understand why I wanted to see her lab work. She was tired, frustrated, angry with her body, and disgusted with what she saw in the mirror. After Joanne told me her story, completed the checklist of symptoms, and jotted down her weight and family medical histories, I had a sense of what she was up against. Her blood work confirmed it.

Joanne was not making mistakes with her diet or exercise plan. At some time over the past few years, Joanne's body began to show the progressive symptoms of Metabolism B. She no longer processed carbohydrate as she once did, and her weight had escalated.

JOANNE'S CLUES

- Midline fat
- Couldn't lose weight on her tried-and-true diets
- Decreased calories and increased physical activity but no weight loss
- Hypoglycemia
- Mother with prediabetes and a sister with gestational diabetes
- Craving for carbohydrates
- Fatigue and mild depression
- Short fuse and irritability

Joanne began the Metabolism Miracle that day. She crossed her fingers as she left my office and I told her that there was no need for luck this time. The program would work.

Eight weeks later, she returned for her first follow-up glowing, in new jeans and a form-fitting top. Her body had lost its excess layer of fat and the belly bulge was gone. She had energy, felt healthy, and looked great. Joanne continues to live the Metabolism Miracle lifestyle and maintains her desired weight!

That sounds fine, you say, for someone who has the luxury of dedicating so much time to her eating patterns and exercise regimen. But what about someone whose schedule makes flexibility impossible? What about someone who works full-time and travels frequently?

MICHAEL: CHANGING THE FUTURE

Michael, a fifty-one-year-old traveling businessman, had just been diagnosed with type 2 diabetes when his assistant called my office, on a doctor's suggestion, to set up an appointment ASAP to "get this thing under control."

Michael arrived frazzled and distracted. His cell phone rang incessantly and he kept checking his wristwatch as he curtly answered my questions. As we went through his history, Michael finally made eye contact and began to tell his story. Although his mother had tried hard and had listened to her physician's direction regarding her dietary intake and medications, she never had good control of her blood sugar. Michael had watched his beloved mother lose her vision and kidney function, and eventually reside in a nursing home, totally dependent on others for her care and enduring kidney dialysis three days a week. She had recently died of complications from type 2 diabetes. Michael wiped his eyes several times as he told this story. "I don't want to end up like my mother," he said.

Michael worked long hours, traveled for business, ate many of his meals in restaurants, and wasn't Betty Crocker in the kitchen. He was divorced and lived alone. He was exhausted, frustrated, annoyed with this diagnosis, and felt he didn't have the time or energy to turn it around.

At five foot ten and 230 pounds, Michael did not exercise. Even with his medication for hypertension and cholesterol, his blood pressure was slightly elevated and his cholesterol/triglycerides exceeded the normal range. When the doctor handed Michael a prescription for oral medication for diabetes, he mentioned that the other medications would soon be increased. Michael hated the idea of more. He was disgusted with his expanding belly and he disliked the person he had become—irritable, nasty, short-tempered, and so very tired.

A diagnosis of type 2 diabetes immediately identified Michael as having Metabolism B. But he had plenty of other clues as well.

MICHAEL'S CLUES

- General overweight and midline fat
- Elevated cholesterol/triglycerides
- Hypertension
- Type 2 diabetes
- Mother with type 2 diabetes
- Feeling anxious, frazzled, irritable
- Being easily distracted
- Fatigue

I asked Michael to keep an open mind and listen to what he needed to do to regain and maintain good health, peace of mind, and lots of energy. I explained the physiology of type 2 diabetes and how this program would, most likely, help to control his blood sugar without medication. I explained how the Metabolism Miracle would decrease the fat around his middle and the fat circulating in his blood vessels, decrease his medications, and fit well into his chaotic lifestyle. He could still eat out and there was no need for him to take cooking lessons!

Michael could adapt each step of the Metabolism Miracle diet to his lifestyle. We planned portable snacks, quick meals, and restaurant meals. For exercise, he would spend a half hour briskly walking back and forth to the train station.

After eight weeks of excellent blood sugar results without medication, a weight loss of 10 pounds, and his physician already considering a decrease in his cholesterol medication, Michael saw a bright prognosis for long-term health and realized he would not have to live a difficult or complicated lifestyle.

It's been more than two years since that initial appointment, and Michael looks and feels great. He continues to follow the maintenance phase of the Miracle and, over the years, he has referred many friends and clients to the Nutrition Center to "get their act together."

THIS IS YOU

You now know that your metabolism is different. You will no longer try to fit a square peg into a round hole because the Metabolism Miracle is a lifetime lifestyle plan that is right for your metabolism. It will help you to lose weight, keep it off, and improve your emotional and physical well-being with as little medication as possible.

You may have been frustrated by weight gain for too long, your lab numbers may be abnormal, and you may have several serious health diagnoses, but that will all improve with the Miracle. Follow the program carefully and you will feel your body begin to change within a week. In as little as eight weeks, you will see major improvements in your weight as well as your physical, emotional, and mental health.

UNDERSTANDING YOUR
UNIQUE METABOLISM

I want to assure you that the Metabolism Miracle is not just another low-carb diet. Every other low-carb diet was written for the general public as a means to lose weight and, in some cases, decrease blood lipids. You can never achieve permanent weight loss on standard low-carb diets that haphazardly introduce the amount, type, and timing of carbohydrates. Standard low-carb diets used by those with metabolism B cause weight regain as soon as carbohydrate is reintroduced.

Unlike other low-carb diets, the three steps of the Metabolism Miracle program were designed to *retrain* your body to process carbohydrate normally rather than overreacting to it. Before you begin the program, it will help to understand how your metabolism differs and causes you to struggle with weight and related health conditions.

Think of your weight and any related health issues as the offshoots of a weed. If you simply treat the offshoots with diet restrictions and medications but don't get to the root, the weed will grow back, often even stronger.

Metabolism B causes your body to overreact to carbohydrate by releasing excess insulin, a fat storage hormone. Too much insulin causes excess fat storage in both the blood (in the form of cholesterol and triglycerides) and the body (in the form of that roll of fat around your middle). The roots of your weight and medical problems include excess insulin release, resistance to your own insulin, and an overreaction to blood sugar. Once you destroy the root, the offshoots—weight, cholesterol, hypertension, and blood sugar issues—will wither away and stay under control with little to no medication.

Although other diets may succeed for a short period of time, they can't maintain weight loss because they fail to work with your body's reaction to carbohydrate. *The* Metabolism Miracle is written to get to the root and retrain your body to process carbohydrate in a normal way.

Knowing exactly what is different about your body is half the battle. The other half is in learning how to treat this difference. That's where the Metabolism Miracle program comes in and empowers you to work with your body instead of against it.

A BAGEL IN THE LIFE OF METABOLISMS A AND B

To understand how Metabolism B reacts to carbohydrates, let's compare you with a friend who has Metabolism A.

You and your friend plan to spend the day shopping. On your way to the mall, you decide to stop for a bagel and coffee. A bagel contains carbohydrate, so as it digests it turns into glucose that is released into the bloodstream. The brain detects this rise in blood glucose and instructs the pancreas to release the right amount of insulin to help bring the blood glucose back into the normal range. Glucose above the normal range will be used to refill glycogen stores in the muscle cells (the stores that you use to move, exercise, and even breathe) and fat cells (the stores that you burn when your muscle and liver stores have been depleted).

Think of insulin as the key that opens the cells' door to allow glucose to enter. Your friend's pancreas released just enough insulin to keep her blood glucose in the normal range, replenish the liver and the muscle cells, and store any excess in fat cells. After eating her bagel, your friend feels full and will remain satisfied during the four to five hours that this process takes.

Your pancreas, however, because of Metabolism B, releases excess insulin to deal with the bagel's glucose rush. Once this insulin helps to refill the glycogen stores in your muscle and liver, the excess keys will open excess fat cells. In an effort to feed these fat cells, you will dip into your normal blood sugar, leaving too little glucose left in the bloodstream to keep up your energy and sense of satiation. Your blood glucose has now dipped below the normal range.

And so, after eating exactly the same meal, you will end up "fatter" than your friend and with lower blood glucose than she has! Your brain senses the low blood glucose and you will begin to feel tired, washed out, and hungry. This all happens only two hours after eating. You look at your friend—she feels great with no fatigue or hunger. What a woman!

You feel the urge for a chocolate bar *now*! Your brain has caused you to crave carbohydrates, the one type of food that will *quickly* bring blood glucose up to normal. You start to feel a bit lightheaded, empty, and irritable. Meanwhile, your friend shops away merrily.

If you cave in and eat that bar, you will immediately feel better, but only for a short time. The carbohydrates contained in the bar will return your blood glucose to normal and relieved, you will think to yourself, *This is the best chocolate bar on earth!* You accuse yourself of being a carboholic. But although you may appear to be out of control, gobbling carbs even as you desperately desire to lose weight, you are really a person following the direction of your brain to bring your blood glucose into a reasonable range.

The satisfaction only lasts a short time. When the chocolate bar digests and your blood sugar begins to rise, your brain once again calls upon your pancreas and once again your pancreas, in its Metabolism B mode, releases too much insulin. The cycle has repeated itself and excess fat cells receive the glucose while your blood glucose levels again dip. You are slowly becoming fatter and, to add insult to injury, the insulin receptors on your fat cells are stretching making it more difficult to open the cells (see "The Key to Insulin Resistance," page 27). Your energy level is dropping again, and you will soon need lunch.

You don't want to ask your friend to stop for lunch already. What if you simply ignore your brain and refuse to give in and eat? What if you remain steadfast and ignore your cravings? Will you be thinner if you ignore carb cravings? Surprisingly, the answer for people with Metabolism B is no.

THE BEAST WITHIN

The human body has a built-in survival mechanism that adds to the challenges of people with Metabolism B and thwarts the weight loss you hope to achieve as you skip a meal. When blood glucose drops to the low end of normal and you choose not to eat, your liver can feed the body.

The body has a five-hour clock that runs continually, day and night. Each time you eat carbohydrate, your body can run on that blood sugar for about five hours. If you choose not to eat within five hours, your liver will release stored blood glucose called *glycogen* that will push blood levels back into the normal range. Releases of liver glycogen keep your body working until you choose to eat again.

If you have ever gone to bed hungry and the next morning you wake up no longer hungry, you are feeling the effects of the self-feeding response. Similarly, if you work through lunch without eating, you might feel hungry for a little while and then the hunger passes. Your liver took care of you by releasing glycogen to raise your blood glucose and satisfy the brain.

When you and your friend decided to postpone lunch, you both passed the five-hour mark and your livers released glycogen. But your friend with Metabolism A releases the right amount of insulin whereas your body overreleases insulin and then ferries the liver's sugar from your bloodstream into your fat cells. You will actually gain weight because you did not eat within five hours!

As a result of that hyper–insulin response, you feel exhausted and irritable. You are developing a midline paunch, your blood pressure and cholesterol may be rising, and you may be crossing the boundary into the tricky waters of diabetes. You constantly struggle with bouts of low

THE KEY TO INSULIN RESISTANCE

You know now that your plumped up fat cells and weight gain come from the hyper–insulin release that characterizes metabolism B. But people with metabolism B have another challenge as well.

Imagine that insulin is a key that must fit perfectly into a keyhole to open a lock. If the keyhole is misshapen, the key can no longer fit. With metabolism B, as fat cells grow in size, their keyholes change shape until the insulin keys can no longer fit to open the cell door, a condition called *insulin resistance*. Blood sugar remains in the bloodstream and as a result, the pancreas works harder than ever to release more insulin that will fit the keyholes, all to no avail. You've eaten, but your cells aren't being "fed" and you end up feeling tired, depressed, fatigued, and very hungry.

A person with "normal" metabolism A has keyholes that can never change, no matter how fat or how thin he or she becomes. Regardless of how large a metabolism A person's fat cells become, insulin keys will always fit the insulin receptor keyholes and will always open the cell to receive the glucose. With metabolism A, a 350-pound man's insulin will fit his insulin receptors as perfectly as it did when he weighed 200 pounds.

When insulin resistance is left untreated, the fatigued pancreas can no longer release enough insulin and much of the insulin that it does release can't fit the keyholes. Continuously facing the locked doors, blood glucose backs up in the bloodstream. This is the beginning of type 2 diabetes and explains why it's so important to use the Metabolism Miracle to get this problem under control before it turns into an irreversible health challenge.

blood sugar that have turned you into a carbohydrate addict. No wonder your self-esteem has plummeted and you feel out of control!

It may not seem fair but your overactive pancreas and resistance to insulin will increase your appetite, weight, and related health issues while wreaking havoc on your life. That is, until you learn to work with it rather than against it.

You haven't gained weight because you've eaten too much fat, sugar, or calories. You've gained weight because your body releases excess insulin, which opens excess fat cells. Those fat cells are fed at the expense of your normal blood sugar, and that depletes your energy level. Of course, you crave more food as a result! You haven't caused these problems but you *can* improve and even correct them. The three steps of the Metabolism Miracle will help you to do it.

You may or may not have heard your doctor mention insulin resistance when assessing your blood glucose. Remember, that the longer someone has lived with the switched on Metabolism B, the more progressive that person's health problems become. Most people know that they weigh much more than they should, given what they eat, and that they can't lose weight and keep it off, and that they feel awful and may be getting sicker. But they may not know they have insulin resistance, metabolic syndrome, and/or a host of other maladies that are related to their alternative metabolism. Insulin resistance is only one of many symptoms that characterize Metabolism B.

THE BAGEL BOMB

Depending upon your metabolism, a bagel can cause two very different reactions in the body. This chart illustrates how the paths diverge.

You and your friend both eat a bagel.

↓

The bagel's carbohydrate turns to blood glucose and enters the bloodstream.

↓

The brain senses the blood glucose rise and instructs the pancreas to release the hormone insulin.

↙   ↘

METABOLISM A
AND THE BAGEL

The pancreas releases exactly the right amount of insulin to handle the rise in blood glucose.

↓

Insulin acts like a key and opens the right amount of fat and muscle cells and returns the glucose in the bloodstream to normal.

↓

Glucose from the bagel provides immediate energy, replaces glycogen in muscle and liver, and any excess is stored as fat.

↓

Equilibrium results in the body feeling satisfied and full after the meal.

↓

Satisfaction lasts for four to five hours until hunger naturally occurs..

METABOLISM B (YOU)
AND THE BAGEL

The pancreas overreacts and releases excess insulin to handle the rise in blood glucose.

↓

Excess insulin opens excess fat cells, ushers in the glucose and leaves too little glucose in the blood for basic energy. Your fat cells get microscopically larger and receptors "stretch" a bit.

↓

The brain signals you to eat more carbohydrate to quickly raise the blood glucose. You feel hungry, tired, shaky, nauseated, and irritable until you eat a carbohydrate snack.

↓

You temporarily feel better as blood glucose rises.

↓

Your brain senses a rise in blood glucose and tells the pancreas to once again release insulin.

↓

Your pancreas overreleases again and the cycle repeats itself.

"TROUBLE TRIGGERS": A GUIDE TO DECIPHERING WHEN AND WHY METABOLISM B PROGRESSED

Until your Metabolism B progressed to the point that symptoms kicked in, your body appeared to respond to food like everyone else's and most reasonable diets worked for you. At some point, however, your metabolism seemed to change. You were born with this genetic predisposition or potential for excess insulin release, insulin resistance, and resultant glucose issues, but for a good chunk of your life, you coasted along without a clue. Although we don't know exactly why the symptoms progress research indicates that certain events may help set off the progression of Metabolism B.

Triggers that may be responsible for the onset of Metabolism B's symptoms include:

1. *Hormonal change.* Growth spurts, puberty, pregnancy, and menopause all cause dramatic hormonal shifts in your body.
2. *Stress.* Stressful challenges involved with adolescence, the college years, entering the adult workforce, marriage, children, career, divorce, death of a loved one, or aging may trigger Metabolism B.
3. *Illness and pain.* A bad flu, virus, surgery, back injury, broken bones, childbirth, severe arthritis, fibromyalgia, cancer, or chronic illness often appear to be the catalyst for Metabolism B's progression.
4. *Medications.* Certain medications for high blood pressure, such as beta blockers as well as steroids such as cortisone and prednisone, can cause increases in blood glucose.
5. *Overweight.* The strain of excess body fat and increasing insulin resistance can tax the body's responses.

6. *Physical Inactivity.* Exercise helps to decrease blood sugar and insulin release.

THE TIMELINE OF METABOLISM B

Now that you know of Metabolism B, it's helpful to look back over your life and assess when the symptoms for alternate metabolism came to the surface.

Put a check next to the time when your metabolism appeared to shift gears and you'll find that from that point on your weight issues, symptoms, and medical history began to change.

- As a child, you were either painfully thin or had a pudgy roll around the tummy. There was no "average" weight in your childhood.
- Despite your being pencil thin or slightly chubby as a child, your weight changed during your teens or midtwenties. You could no longer get away with dietary indiscretions and could gain five pounds in one weekend! You noticed that although you ate less than your friends, you were always heavier than they.
- After childbirth, women with Metabolism B report extreme frustration losing weight. After each delivery, weight loss becomes even more difficult.
- Women who haven't had children may notice a change in their weight irrespective of childbirth. They may feel stressed, overwhelmed, and rushed with less time for exercise and relaxation.
- Men may notice that they begin to develop a midline paunch. Later, they have difficulty buttoning their bottom shirt button and their waist size begins to increase from 32 to 34 to 36 and

up. Work and family obligations take precedence over time spent working out.

- Eventually, weight-loss methods that successfully knocked off five or ten pounds in the past stopped working. The older you got, the harder it became to lose weight. At some point, you seemed to lose the battle and cross the line and give up.

- No matter what diet program you tried, your excess weight never came off and stayed off. Your friends made diet changes and got results; you made the same changes and gained weight!

- Your overall health began to change and you needed medication for weight-related health problems. You decided to buy a pill box!

- You began to feel much older than your age. Your face looked puffy and there were bags under your eyes. You felt bloated, especially after eating a meal, and you needed to unbutton your jeans to breathe. You began to feel a variety of aches and pains and you felt tapped of energy. Mild depression and bouts of anxiety entered your life. You slept fitfully and woke up tired.

- Your carbohydrate addiction got worse. You opened the kitchen cabinets and went from bag to carton, bingeing on carb foods. After opening a bag of chips or cookies, you kept returning for more than you intended. You began to worry that you had lost control. Why did you lack the willpower?

The Common Eating Habits
of Metabolism B

Over the years I've met thousands of people with Metabolism B. When they sit down in my office to tell their story, it always amazes me how many eating habits they share. See if you recognize yourself in any of these common descriptions.

- Very often, the first point that my patients want to convey is that they don't eat the amount of food that should equal the weight on the scale. Doctors and nutritionists have accused them of underreporting food consumption, closet eating, purging, or outright lying on their diet recall!
- People with Metabolism B have a history of yo-yo dieting and can recall losing and regaining hundreds of pounds throughout their lifetime. They feel frustrated, ashamed, and despondent.
- The breakfast bomb: Half of these patients aren't hungry in the morning and cannot possibly eat breakfast. The other half cannot function without eating in the morning. It's all or nothing regarding the first meal of the day!
- Those who do eat breakfast crave carbohydrates. They seek combinations of toast, bagels, orange juice, cereal with milk, Danishes, muffins, doughnuts, and fruited yogurt.
- They feel that they are in "their best control" before they eat anything for the day. They report feeling hungrier once they begin to eat.
- Metabolism B patients often report needing to eat two or three hours after a meal. Midmorning, late afternoon, and nighttime cravings and snacking are very common. When they hold off on eating they may get cranky, nauseated, or lightheaded.
- After lunch, people with Metabolism B frequently feel drowsy and need a nap. They also report craving chocolate, a salty/crunchy snack, or caffeine in the afternoon.
- Most patients with Metabolism B relate needing a caffeine "lift" in the morning or late afternoon. They drink coffee, tea, iced tea, caffeinated soft drinks, energy drinks, or chocolate to pick up their energy.

The Common Eating Habits of Metabolism B *(continued)*

- Although they'd like to prepare a balanced dinner, these individuals list demanding careers, dual-career families, family commitments, and fatigue among the reasons that they dine out or bring in dinner. Many report having pizza, Chinese food, deli food, fast food, or take-out dinners at least twice a week.
- When eating out, most of these patients try to ignore the bread basket but once they begin sampling it, they have a difficult time controlling their consumption of bread and rolls.
- Most don't eat dessert as part of dinner but seem to have a "craving" for sweets in the course of the evening. Ice cream is a favorite nighttime snack.
- Pasta can cause a major problem for the Metabolism B patient. Most admit to eating several full plates for the meal, snitching some as they clear the table, picking at the pasta in the refrigerator throughout the evening, and even digging into the pasta bowl in the morning.
- Many people with Metabolism B feel fixated on food, daydreaming about it throughout their day and even thinking about what they are going to eat for dinner as they eat their breakfast.
- Many report sleepiness after eating their nighttime meal and falling asleep in a chair watching the evening news. They wake up a little later in the evening, starving, and begin their nighttime snacking.
- A significant number wake up hungry in the middle of the night. Some get out of bed and head to the refrigerator at 2:00 or 3:00 a.m. for a snack.
- Almost every Metabolism B patient I counsel reports eating more when he/she is under stress. These patients typically can't stop snacking when they are stressed.

Interestingly, when your Metabolism B is correctly treated, the eating patterns that were your way of life lessen or even disappear. People cannot believe that the foods they used to crave and look forward to eating no longer have that effect on them. It turns out that the food wasn't that "delicious"; it just provided the necessary blood glucose boost and literally gave comfort. When blood sugar stays in the normal zone, without peaks and valleys, these foods become like any other food.

WHAT HAPPENED? "OTHER DIETS USED TO WORK FOR ME"

By now you have a good understanding of how Metabolism B directs your body to store excess blood sugar into your fat cells. The Metabolism Miracle will help to temper your pancreas, calming the insulin release and fat production so that permanent weight loss can occur. But why wouldn't any diet help you to lose weight?

When your friends with Metabolism A want to lose weight, they can follow any reasonable diet because their metabolism follows the classic formula found in any basic nutrition textbook:

$$\text{Calories eaten} - \text{calories burned} = \text{weight}$$

In other words, your friends who have metabolism A will gain weight if they consume more calories than they burn off. But they will lose weight if they cut back on total calories while increasing their physical activity. Your friends' cholesterol is determined by their weight, physical activity, and intake of fatty foods. Their triglycerides may increase because of excess alcohol or certain medications, or their blood pressure may increase from excess weight or sensitivity to sodium. However, your weight, cholesterol, triglycerides, blood pressure, and blood sugar are all linked to hormonal imbalance and excess fat storage.

You now know that your metabolism is very different. The law of calories doesn't apply to people with Metabolism B. You may eat far fewer calories than your friends and lose weight initially but because your body stores excess blood sugar as fat, a diet based on calories will never work for you long term. Your weight, midline fat, and cholesterol are not entirely the result of excess calories or inadequate physical activity. They are caused by the hypermetabolism of carbohydrate and blood glucose being stored excessively in fat cells.

"HELP ME, DOC!"

Most people with Metabolism B have been told by their physician, "You need to lose twenty pounds"—or even more. Naturally, you are very aware that you need to lose twenty pounds, but, despite all of your attempts, you can't seem to make it happen. If you have hypertension you hear, "Cut down on salt and lose some weight." When your cholesterol rises, you hear, "Reduce fats and lose some weight." If you progress to diabetes, the advice changes only slightly: "Watch your sugar intake and lose some weight." Unfortunately, that's the extent of the nutrition advice that many patients hear. They leave their doctor's office with a handful of prescriptions, a diet sheet, and a follow-up appointment date. The doctor doesn't have the key to successful weight loss for people with Metabolism B.

In an effort to get some answers, some patients seek out a registered dietitian (RD) and leave that appointment with a copy of the same 1,500-calorie low-fat/low-cholesterol/low-salt playbook that the RD uses for everyone in your condition. But all these patients' hard work to follow the directions from both their doctor and nutritionist yields little weight loss. Why? Because, if they have Metabolism B, this standard diet, based on "calories in" minus "calories out," will never work for them!

MISGUIDED GUIDELINES

The medical community has known for at least twenty years that many of us have this combination of symptoms that make up what I refer to as Metabolism B. They include difficulty losing weight, overrelease of insulin, blood sugar problems, insulin resistance, metabolic syndrome, high cholesterol and blood pressure, fatigue, depression, carb cravings, and more. And although books have been written to address specific symptoms—diets for insulin resistance or metabolic syndrome, for example—no one has combined the symptoms to successfully tackle them as a group. This is how *The Metabolism Miracle* differs from every other weight-loss book currently available.

None of the medical associations responsible for setting diet guidelines have yet to adapt an effective diet and lifestyle plan for the population with Metabolism B. Meanwhile, the old diet guidelines may end up harming rather than improving the weight and health of people with this alternative metabolism.

Please understand that the foundations for traditional diet guidelines were laid before Metabolism B had been identified. They were, in fact, the very guidelines that I depended upon to counsel my patients before I researched the basis for my Metabolism Miracle program. Now that we understand Metabolism B, it astounds me how misguided some of the medical establishment's guidelines continue to be.

Everyone recognizes the USDA food pyramid with its base of starches and grains. But think about it—that bottom-heavy section encourages us to choose more than half of our daily food from *carbohydrate*! For years, the American Diabetes Association has recommended that between 50 to 55 percent of calories consumed daily by people with diabetes (all of whom have Metabolism B) should come in the form of *carbohydrate*! The American Medical Association and the American Heart Association recommend low-fat/low-cholesterol diets (by nature higher in *carbohydrate*) for *anyone* with heart disease.

This type of carbohydrate-dense diet logic made sense when we thought that only Metabolism A existed. But we now know that a large portion of the population, including the majority of people with diabetes and heart disease, has Metabolism B and, unless they work with their bodies to handle carbohydrate normally, they store much of their blood sugar as fat rather than use it as energy. No wonder patients with heart disease who follow low-fat/low-cholesterol diets can rarely get their lipids to decrease and must instead depend on statins and other medications to control hypertension and cholesterol.

Recommending that people with Metabolism B, who have trouble processing carbohydrate, consume at least half of their calories from carbohydrate is like advising people with an allergy to dairy to consume half of their daily calories from dairy foods!

For someone with Metabolism B, a higher carb diet causes cholesterol, triglycerides, blood pressure, and weight to increase! If people with Metabolism B follow these misguided guidelines without first correcting their overreaction to carb, their pancreas will churn out excess insulin and may even begin to tire. They will gain weight, may require increased doses of medication, and many will become prediabetic or even develop type 2 diabetes. Look around you—the country really is becoming heavier and sicker.

THE "CARB IS A CARB" MYTH

Perhaps you've heard the mantra, "A carb is a carb." It is the basis for yet another dietary myth. This is the theory behind carbohydrate

WHY OTHER DIETS HAVE FAILED YOU

You probably have a long history of trying diets that work for a while but ultimately fail to keep weight at bay, no matter how closely you follow the rules. The bottom line is that Metabolism B won't respond to the traditional formula for weight loss, which depends upon eating fewer calories than you burn off in a day. This list explains why these popular diets fail anyone with Metabolism B.

Traditional Weight-Loss Program: This approach, based on decreasing the calories you consume while increasing the calories you burn, cannot work for those with Metabolism B because their weight is determined in great part by their response to carbohydrate and blood sugar rise, not simply calories in/calories out.

Low-Fat and Low-Cholesterol Diets: When you restrict fat grams, you automatically restrict many protein foods such as red meat, cheese, and peanut butter. With restrictions of both protein and fat, carbohydrate is left to fill the gap. For people with Metabolism B, excess carbohydrate stimulates excess insulin that then stores the carbohydrate glucose as fat. Imagine struggling to follow a low-fat and low-cholesterol diet and watching your cholesterol rise!

Low-Carb Diet Program: Although low-carb diets can often produce an initial weight loss, when carbohydrate is reintroduced, without regard to amount, type, or timing, a Metabolism B dieter immediately overreacts to the blood sugar rise and weight gain is almost instantaneous. Also, a typical low-carb diet does not completely rest the liver from self-feeding every five hours. (See "The Beast Within," page 26). As a result, when you limit carb or skip a meal, the liver still step up to the plate and releases glycogen stores for energy. For those with Metabolism B, the pancreas will overrespond with insulin to enable excess glucose to enter fat cells and generate weight gain!

Very Low-Calorie Diet (VLCD): These medically supervised liquid diets, containing only 500 to 800 calories per day, put the body into a starvation mode. After an initial weight loss, your brain perceives that it is getting too few calories to maintain normal life functions and keep you alive, so it slows metabolic rate to preserve every morsel you consume. At the same time, the Metabolism B pancreas continues to overrespond to blood sugar from carbohydrates and from the liver's release of glycogen. As soon as the dieter reverts to even a low 1,000 calories (most people need more than 1,400 calories), his or her weight begins to balloon.

Fad Diets: Diets that focus on magic potions such as cabbage soup, grapefruit, crackers and water, chocolate, or foods of one color will not work for anyone long term. But you already knew that, right?

counting, which maintains that every carbohydrate gram you eat will eventually turn into blood sugar and so . . ."a carb is a carb." This misconception has wreaked havoc for people with Metabolism B and is one of the reasons that traditional carb-counting diets will not work for people with alternative metabolism.

To illustrate the theory consider that both one slice of whole wheat toast and two regular-size chocolate chip cookies contain 15 grams of carbohydrate. Carbohydrate counting asserts that you may choose the carbohydrates you need from *any* category: fruit, milk, starch, or

THE WAKE-UP CALL

Sometimes people who have followed all of their doctor's advice and look like the picture of health have a frightening wake-up call. That's when understanding that they have Metabolism B becomes a matter of life or death.

George loves life. He has been married for over thirty years and has a grandson with whom he enjoys fishing. The fifty-seven-year-old works hard and looks forward to retirement when he plans to read, walk, fish, and fish—the man loves to fish!

He saw his cardiologist yearly for high cholesterol, walked daily, took his prescribed medications, and followed his low-fat/low-cholesterol diet. When he grilled, he used superlean sirloin, skinless chicken, and fish. He snacked on fat-free pretzels and whole-grain crackers. His potato salad was fat free and he used frozen fruit bars for dessert. He was determined, despite his high cholesterol, to watch his first grandchild grow up.

But two years ago a heart attack shook up his world.

No one expected cardiac problems in a man who was so careful, so cautious, and so health-conscious. He entered my office scared, explaining that he didn't know what else he could possibly do to prevent another heart attack.

I listened to George's story and took a good look at this man who had followed the traditional diet guidelines to a T. He had a roll of fat around his middle despite daily exercise and his diet. He took medications for blood pressure, cholesterol, acid reflux, and anxiety. He complained of fatigue and feeling sleepy after meals. He told me that over the past few years he didn't feel like himself, that something felt "off."

sweets. According to the theory, your blood sugar will rise equally after you consume either the whole grain toast or the cookies. The problem with this philosophy is that different carbohydrates change into blood sugar at different speeds and with different intensities.

When you eat the two cookies, your blood sugar will immediately increase with a sharp spike. By contrast, the whole wheat toast, or any carbohydrate that is naturally high in fiber and low in added sugar, will change to blood sugar at a slower speed without the intense spike.

The Wake-Up Call *(continued)*

He couldn't sleep well, he woke up tired, and although he loved his wife, his libido had declined. In fact, his level of joy had also decreased. He couldn't keep up with his grandson and he even admitted to being less interested in fishing!

His father had died of a heart attack at the age of sixty and George's own lab report was telling: his glucose was 112 (normal is 65–99 mg/dL [3.6–5.5 mmol/L]), and his LDL cholesterol, triglycerides, and blood pressure were all higher than normal. In fact, he was prediabetic without knowing it.

I explained that the low-fat/low-cholesterol diet was high in the carbohydrate that probably caused his alternative metabolism to overprocess blood glucose into fat. The diet he had so faithfully followed was working against him and may even have been a contributing factor to his heart attack.

George was so entrenched in the low-fat/low-cholesterol diet that he found it difficult to shift gears. His lean protein choices and heart-healthy fat intake were a perfect backdrop for the Miracle program, but he had to make adjustments to his intake of carbohydrates. He was a desperate man and he wanted his future and life back.

Eight weeks after he began the Metabolism Miracle, George returned, having lost four inches of fat off his belly. His blood pressure, LDL cholesterol, and triglycerides had all improved. He felt energetic and confident and was thrilled with the ease of the program. He left the office with a spring in his step and told me that his fishing pole was already in his car!

Low-impact carbohydrates, such as brown rice or whole-grain bread, for example, have more staying power; they do not prompt the pancreas to release a quick flood of insulin. Instead, their slower release of blood sugar prompts a slower release of insulin. In the medical world, a carbohydrate's impact is determined by its *glycemic index*, which rates how rapidly a carb turns into glucose. In *The Metabolism Miracle*, we'll simply tag carbohydrates with the terms *low impact* and *high impact*.

You can see how "a carb is a carb" myth becomes a problem. When someone with Metabolism B chooses high-impact carbs, such as cookies, in their diet, they tax their insulin response much more than if they were to eat exactly the same number of carbohydrates but in a low-impact form, such as the whole wheat bread.

When you have Metabolism B, you must toss out the old carbohydrate myths to achieve permanent weight loss and avoid health issues down the road. It took me a long time to figure out how to save myself from the black hole of textbook diets but, like my patients who have followed the Metabolism Miracle program, I have kept off weight, improved my health and well-being, and now have boundless energy.

PART TWO

A 3-Step Plan to Weight Loss That Will Stay Off

STEP ONE—CARB REHAB: EIGHT WEEKS TO A NEW LIFE

STEP-ONE BASICS

Time: 8 weeks

The challenge: A low-carb period to rest your overworked pancreas and liver while shrinking fat cells

Results: Your energy will soar and you'll feel content. You will lose weight and your belly fat will slim down. Meanwhile, cholesterol, triglycerides, blood sugar, and blood pressure all decrease.

Think of Step One of the Metabolism Miracle as spring cleaning. You will eat many of your favorite foods in this easy, straightforward step but you will also, in essence, clean up the metabolic mess that has taken control of your body.

For the eight weeks of Step One, you will cut out most carbohydrates from your diet. This will give your pancreas a long-overdue vacation so that it can regroup and reprogram to handle carbohydrates healthily. As you rest your overworked system, your body will create a clean slate for a future at the weight that you look and feel your best.

As a registered dietitian, I was never a fan of low-carb diets. I felt that there was something wrong with eliminating an entire group of nutrients from the daily diet. Carbohydrate is the preferred fuel for the body. So how could eliminating it be healthy?

After years of researching Metabolism B, I changed my mind. As it turns out, there is only one way to nonmedically control the blood glucose imbalance that plagues people with this alternative metabolism. The program must *temporarily* eliminate most carbohydrates from the diet. This rehabilitative state accomplishes two things:

1. By eliminating carb-dense foods, *you* stop contributing sugar to your bloodstream.
2. The temporary elimination of most carbs will enable the liver to deplete most of the glycogen stores it uses for the self-feeding mechanism.

As a result, for the first eight weeks of Step One, your blood sugar will run smoothly, with no spikes that would stimulate the pancreas to overrelease insulin. Your pancreas and liver will take a much-needed temporary vacation to rest and rejuvenate.

A very low-carb diet is not nutritionally balanced but, as a *temporary* choice to reset a healthy metabolism, it works well by deliberately leaving the pancreas and liver in a state of rest. Carbs come back into the picture on Steps Two and Three, but by then you have established a new metabolic balance that your body can work with beautifully.

THE THREE-DAY KICKER

By the fourth day of Step One, you will be delighted with the changes that your body feels. But the first three days of Step One will be tough—the very reason I've nicknamed this step "rehab" or "detox." Realize that your body has been using carbohydrate for fuel since the day you were born. Now, you are asking your brain to choose an alternative fuel source for a short time. Give yourself a few days to acclimate to this new approach. Rome wasn't built in a day.

For the first three days, you can expect to feel tired, cranky, hungry (even as you eat plenty of food), carb-crazed, slightly shaky, lightheaded, and a little headachy. Hold on—*you can do it.*

After three days, you will begin to feel much better with more energy, no hunger, and no carb cravings. You will also be less irritable and much more relaxed. Within a week, once this step is in full swing, you will have no carb cravings and your friends and family will probably mention how pleasant you are to be around.

Why are those first three days so difficult? Recall that your liver contains a three-day stockpile of blood sugar in the form of glycogen. When you begin Step One and cut out dense carbohydrate from your diet, your liver will feed you with a meal's worth of glycogen around the clock every five hours. That's almost five meals per day! In response to each of those meals, your pancreas will overrelease insulin and your blood sugar will continue to roller-coaster even though you will not be eating much carb. Those blood sugar highs and lows will initially make you irritable and cranky.

At the end of Step One's first three days, as you continue to eliminate blatant carbohydrates and your liver remains purposely depleted of most of its glycogen stores, your brain will have to come up with an alternative plan for fueling the body. As long as you continue to eliminate carbs and your liver remains depleted of glycogen, the brain will choose between consuming muscle or fat for the body's energy needs.

Exercise plays an important role in the Metabolism Miracle as it literally energizes and activates muscle. The brain will leave active muscle cells alone and focus on consuming the inactive fat cells for energy needs.

Step One is setting up the body exactly as we want it for the next eight weeks, to:

- Retain muscle
- Derive energy from fat
- Consume fat circulating as excess cholesterol and triglycerides
- Rest the overworked pancreas and liver

Your metabolism will begin to adjust to a more stable blood sugar and miraculously, your body will consume fat like never before.

To maximize your success and keep yourself in tip-top health, it is important that you follow ten easy guidelines while on the program. Once you weave them into your life and feel the difference that they make, you'll understand why I call them "Rules to Thrive By." See chapter 8 for more on these guidelines.

1. Drink at least 64 ounces of water and caffeine-free fluids daily.
2. Avoid gaps of more than five hours without a meal or snack. Spread your food intake throughout the entire day and even into the night. Within one hour of waking up and right before bed, be sure to have a meal or snack.
3. Take the recommended vitamins, minerals, and supplements.
4. Choose nonnutritive sweeteners with care. I recommend the use of sucralose or stevia as a sugar substitute.

FIND YOUR BASELINE

Before you begin Step One, take stock of what you're starting with by noting your weight and body measurements (chest, waist, hips, and more—see page 169–170 in chapter 10 for specific directions). Try to resist remeasuring or reweighing until the very last day of Step One's eight weeks. You will be spared the frustration of the roller-coaster weight loss that characterizes Metabolism B and you will be ecstatic when you see the final results.

5. Judge the carbohydrate content of packaged foods by reading the
   Nutrition Facts section of food labels and using "the formula."
   (See "Easy Carb Counting," page 54.)
6. Consider drinking green tea daily.
7. Increase your physical activity to include a minimum of 30
   minutes, five times per week.
8. Eat allowed foods liberally, but not to excess.
9. Practice relaxing. Take a few minutes each day to close your eyes,
   breathe deeply, shed your stress, and clear your mind.
10. Think positively! First thing in the morning and the last thing at
    night, remind yourself of your good health, weight loss, high
    energy level, continuing progress, and positive future.

SIMPLE, SIMPLE, SIMPLE

Perhaps the best part about Step One, besides the fat loss and energy
boost, is its ease and simplicity. During Step One, foods fall into two
categories: yes and no. People find these food choices incredibly easy
to make.

Look at the arrow sheet in this chapter. Each of the four arrows represents a category of foods: lean proteins, healthy fats, allowed vegetables, and carbohydrates. During the eight weeks of Step One, you may
eat liberally from the first three arrows but you must avoid the foods in
the carbohydrate arrow. The foods in the protein, fat, and allowed veggie arrows don't require a carb check. You won't need to read food labels for the carb content of nuts, cheese, cottage cheese, or broccoli.
Only the carb-containing foods that are starred or marked "5x5" carbs
require a label check. These foods must be limited to 5 grams in a five-
hour period, and include low-carb bread, low-carb yogurt, low-carb
milk, and the like.

Although most foods contain a combination of nutrients, they are
classified into their arrow by the main nutrient that they contain. For

example, flank steak and chicken fall into the protein arrow, olive oil and nuts fall into the fat arrow, and white potatoes fall into the carbohydrate arrow.

Sometimes, however, foods can be deceptive. Take the two dairy foods cheese and yogurt. Cheese contains mostly protein, so it fits into the protein arrow. Low-fat yogurt contains protein and fat but its main nutrient is carbohydrate, so this dairy product is in the carbohydrate arrow.

Many people are surprised to learn that milk, fruit, carrots, and lentils also fit into the carbohydrate arrow. Foods in the carb arrow will have a dramatic impact on blood sugar and cause your pancreas to quickly release insulin. You must avoid these foods during Step One. Not even a pinch.

There is no need to weigh, measure, count, or plot foods from the lean protein, healthy fat, and vegetable arrows. These foods will not stimulate the insulin roller coaster. You can eat them whenever you wish.

You'll notice a small horizontal arrow labeled "5x5 carbs." Although typical bread, crackers, yogurt, and other carbohydrate-dense foods must be avoided during Step One, the food industry has come up with low-carb versions of these foods that fit sparingly into Step One. I'll explain this on page 56.

Consider hanging a copy of the "Arrow Sheet" on your refrigerator or keeping one at the office or in your bag to remind you of the foods to avoid on Step One and those that you may eat freely.

CARB CONTROL

The key to Step One is carbohydrate control. You won't eliminate all carbohydrate foods from your diet, but you'll temporarily avoid most of them. The foods in the protein, fat, and veggie arrows that are not starred do not require a food label check even though they contain a limited amount of carb.

During any five-hour period of Step One, you may eat 5 grams of carbohydrate. This "5x5 rule" allows you to eat limited carb grams without stimulating your pancreas to release insulin.

Any carbohydrate above the 5-gram ceiling—1/2 cup sugar-free ice cream with its 10 grams of carb, for example—will alert the pancreas to release insulin and will put you right back into the metabolic chaos your body desperately needs to escape. Keep carb intake under the 5-gram bar and your pancreas will remain in its curative resting state.

So how do you know which foods have 5 grams or less of carbohydrates? The list of carbohydrates that you must absolutely avoid during Step One all exceed the 5-gram limit (see Step One "Carbs to Avoid," page 53). But a number of carbohydrate foods can be eaten during Step One. I call these foods "5x5 carbs" because you can tally their carbohydrate total with a quick, easy formula to decide if they fit the 5x5 rule. Any foods that have been starred (*) on the food lists fit into the 5x5 category. You must be the judge. Never rely on marketing ploys used on the package to tell you the number of carb grams the product contains. You must do the math.

YOU CAN DO IT

Almost every patient with Metabolism B in my practice who sees the "Carbs to Avoid List" begins to panic. They grow pale, shake their head, and declare, "There is no way that I can do this for eight weeks!"

Your strong reaction to this list of foods is just one more affirmation that you have Metabolism B. However, you should know that every one of the patients who completed the first three days of Step One, completed the remainder of the eight weeks.

THE
Arrow Sheet

PROTEIN ARROW
YES
For all steps
(Lean, lite, or low-fat preferred)

Meat
Poultry
Fish and shellfish
Cheese
Cottage cheese
Eggs
Egg substitutes

Natural nut butter
Natural seed butter
Tofu
Unsweetened soy milk
Edamame
*Select protein shakes

Although meats and cheeses are primarily protein, they vary tremendously in their fat content. The recommended protein sources in the Metabolism Miracle program will be heart healthy and lean. You can feel free to enjoy them liberally.

NEUTRAL VEGGIES ARROW
YES
For all steps

Artichokes and artichoke hearts
Asparagus
Green or wax beans
Bean sprouts
Broccoli
Brussels sprouts
Cabbage
Cauliflower

Celery
Cucumbers
Dill Pickles
Eggplant
Jicama (max 1 cup)
Onions and scallions
Greens (collards, kale, mustard, turnip, spinach)

Kohlrabi
Leeks
Mushrooms
Okra
Peppers (all varieties)
Lettuce and other salad greens
Radishes
Spaghetti squash

Sauerkraut
Tomatoes (maximum 1 fresh tomato per meal or 10 cherry tomatoes, $\frac{1}{2}$ cup canned tomatoes, $\frac{1}{2}$ cup tomato salsa, 4 oz. tomato/veggie juice)
Turnips
Zucchini and summer squash

FAT ARROW
YES
For all steps
(Lite or low-fat preferred)

Butter
Margarine
Sour cream
Mayonnaise
Cream
Half-and-half

Oil
Salad dressing
Olives
Avocados
Nuts
Seeds
Whipped Cream

CARBOHYDRATE ARROW

(Carbohydrate foods will require label check for Step Two and Three)

Bread
Wraps
Rolls
Buns
Bread Products
Pasta
Rice

Crackers, pretzels, chips
Cereal and granola bars
Cereal (hot or cold)
Other grains
Fruit
Fruit juice
Potatoes and sweet potatoes

Carrots
Parsnips
Beets
Winter squash
Acorn squash
Pumpkin
Milk

Yogurt
Sweetened beverages
Sweets and desserts
Carb-containing foods that fail the 5 gram "counter" test

NO
for Step One

YES for all Steps
* 5 GRAM "COUNTER" CARBS
(Step One: optional at meals and bedtime snacks.
Steps Two and Three: can be added into carb total for a meal/snack on Steps Two and Three.)

* Low-carb bread
* Low-carb tortillas
* Low-carb wraps
* Low-carb crackers
* Low-carb ketchup
* Low-carb yogurts

* Low-carb juices
* Low-carb milk
* Low-carb protein drinks with 2–5 grams net carb
* Foods or recipes in the serving size that provide 5 or less grams net carb

* All of the starred foods must pass the net-carb test and fit the 5 gram "counter" carb rule (page 41).
Net carb grams ≤ 1 gram = neutral

Your body desires to run on carbohydrate but it is built to survive with a mechanism to get you through periods without carb. If there is no carbohydrate, the body will run off the liver's stores of glycogen for three days. On the fourth day, it will begin to burn muscle or fat. Because you will be physically active, the exercise will steer your body to burn fat rather than muscle.

On day four, you will not only shift to fat burning, but your brain will take the edge off the absence of carbohydrates. Imagine you are stranded in the desert without carbohydrates. As long as you continue to avoid carb and stay in the fat-burning mode, your brain will shut down your carb cravings, infuse you with energy, and allow you to think clearly so that you can continue looking for food to survive.

The eight weeks will be a breeze if you follow the 5x5 rule and avoid foods containing more than 5 grams of carbohydrate in a five-hour period. In Step One, you have an option to include a 5-gram net carb at each of your meals, at bedtime, and even in the middle of the night. You can do this without interrupting the new peace that your body has found.

EASY CARB COUNTING

It may sound like work to figure out how many carbohydrates any particular food has, but in fact it's quite simple. An easy formula, the net carb formula, is the only one you will need to use during the three steps of the Metabolism Miracle.

THE NET CARB FORMULA

Total carbohydrate grams – dietary fiber grams = net carb grams

To use it, look at the nutrition facts label on any food. The only numbers you need pay attention to are serving size, total carbohydrate grams, and dietary fiber grams. The words "total carbohydrate" will always be in dark, bold type on the label. Beneath them, in lighter type and slightly indented, you will find "dietary fiber," along with a slew of other terms such as "sugar" and "sugar alcohol."

All of these subcategories are included in the total carb grams. Dietary fiber, however, although included in the total carb grams, will never change into blood sugar and tax the pancreas. Instead, it goes through your digestive system unabsorbed. Subtracting the fiber, then, allows you to see all the carb that does affect your blood sugar and insulin release. That is the *net carb* and it is key to keeping your Metabolism B on track.

Nutrition Facts	
Serving Size 1 cup (228g)	
Servings Per Container 2	
Amount Per Serving	
Calories 260	Calories from fat 120
	% Daily Value*
Total Fat 13g	20%
Saturated Fat 5g	25%
Cholesterol 30mg	10%
Sodium 660mg	28%
Total Carbohydrate 31g	10%
Dietary Fiber 0g	0%
Sugars 5g	
Protein 5g	
Vitamin A 4% • Vitamin C 2%	
Calcium 15% • Iron 4%	

* Percent Daily Values are based on a 2,000 calorie diet. Your daily value may be higher or lower depending on your calorie needs:

	Calories:	2,000	2,500
Total Fat	Less than	65g	80g
Sat Fat	Less than	20g	25g
Cholesterol	Less than	300mg	300mg
Sodium	Less than	2,400mg	2,400mg
Total Carbohydrate		300g	375g
Dietary Fiber		25g	30g

Calories per gram:
Fat 9 • Carbohydrate 4 • Protein 4

HOW TO CALCULATE NET CARBS

Here is an example of how to read a food label and calculate the product's net carbs.

KRAZY KRISPIES CEREAL
SERVING SIZE: 3/4 cup
TOTAL CARBOHYDRATE: 22 grams
DIETARY FIBER: 2 grams

Subtract the dietary fiber (2 grams) from the total carbohydrate (22 grams) and you have the net carbs (20 grams) for a 3/4-cup serving of cereal:

$$22 - 2 = 20$$

total   dietary   net
carb   fiber   carbs

Obviously, with 20 net carbs, this cereal will *not* fit into Step One of the Metabolism Miracle.

Now, let's look at another example:

> **LOW CARB TORTILLA**
> **SERVING SIZE:** 1 tortilla
> **TOTAL CARBOHYDRATE:** 10 grams
> **DIETARY FIBER:** 5 grams

$$10 - 5 = 5$$

total	dietary	net
carb	fiber	carbs

With only 5 net carbs, the tortilla fits into Step One, as long as you remember the 5x5 rule and make it the only carb food you eat in a five-hour period of time.

5x5 Carbs*

Many people miss breads, crackers, and other traditionally high-carbohydrate foods during Step One of the program. You might consider eating specially designed low-carb versions of these foods, such as the tortilla in our second example (see low carb tortilla). But don't trust the carb count on the front of the package. Instead, always use the net carb formula to determine the carbohydrates in a serving, and remember the 5x5 rule. If your low-carb bread comes up at 6 grams of carbohydrate, remove the top crust.

The same goes for a number of starred items in the Step One proteins, fats, and vegetable lists, such as processed peanut butter and prepared salad dressings. You can apply the net carb formula to any foods

---

* The terms *5x5 carbs* and *5 gram "counter" carbs* are used interchangeably in the Metabolism Miracle program.

BUYER BEWARE

Those tempting whole-grain crackers with their "low-carb" label may look like they fit into the 5x5 rule, but watch out. Marketing on the front of packages can be deceptively tricky. Food companies have different definitions of "low carb" and "sugar free," and what fits into one low-carb diet may not fit into the Metabolism Miracle diet.

The only way to determine whether the crackers have 5 grams or less carbohydrate and can fit into Step One is to run a serving size through the net carb formula: Total carb – dietary fiber = net carb.

Serving Size: 6 crackers
Total Carbohydrate: 11 grams
Dietary Fiber: 3 grams

11 – 3 = **8 grams**

These crackers do *not* fit into Step One of the Metabolism Miracle. Keep trying—you'll find another product that you love, which will have 5 grams or less net carb and keep you on the healthy path you've been following.

of which you're unsure, and reduce your serving size accordingly if necessary. The key is simply to stay aware of how many carbohydrates sneak onto your plate.

Unstarred foods in the protein and healthy fat arrow do *not* require a 5x5 check. Since cheese, cottage cheese, and nuts are not starred, you need not check their labels for carb content. Consider them to be liberal foods.

Don't make the mistake of stacking carbohydrate foods within the same five-hour period. The 5x5 applies to five hours elapsed, total, for foods and beverages consumed. If you choose a 5-gram low-carb wrap for lunch at noon and a 3-gram carb-controlled yogurt for a snack at 2:30 p.m., the combined 8 grams of carbohydrate will exceed the 5x5 rule because only two and a half hours have elapsed. The resting pancreas will detect a rise in blood sugar from the 8 grams of carbohydrate and awaken to release insulin, just the outcome you are trying to avoid.

To make life easier, I usually decide if I want a 5x5 or starred carbohydrate at breakfast, lunch, dinner, bedtime, and in the middle of the night. I don't use them for between-meal snacks.

Sugar Shakedown

Did you know that when you see the word *sugar* on a food label, it refers only to sucrose (table sugar)? All other sweeteners in a food—corn syrup, fructose, or honey, for example—are not included in the "sugar" tally. It is not necessary to look at sugar grams as sugar is only one small part of the carbohydrate picture. Total carb grams will show you *all* of the carbs in the food item.

What about Sugar Alcohol?

When reading an ingredient list of products labeled "sugar free," "low sugar," or "low carb," you'll often come across ingredients that end in *ol*, such as mannitol, xylitol, and sorbitol. Ingredients ending in *ol* are most

Size Matters

Be sure to note the serving size, which can trip you up unexpectedly. Take, for instance, a bottle of flavored iced tea. The 12-ounce bottle looks like one serving, but when you check the nutrition facts label you see that it is in fact two and half servings. Unless you check the label, you may innocently gulp down the entire bottle with more than twice the carbs you thought you were drinking.

Creative serving sizes can push all of your hard effort on Step One right off track. Keep your eye on the serving sizes when you use the net carb formula.

likely sugar alcohols. These ingredients are **not** calorie free. They have less impact on blood glucose than actual sugar because they are not completely absorbed in the GI tract. Because they don't fully absorb, sugar alcohol is known to cause bloating, gas, flatulence, and diarrhea.

When you read the Nutrition Facts label, you'll often note "sugar alcohol" under the heading for total carbohydrate. But do not be fooled: Sugar alcohol *does* affect blood sugar and insulin release. It is listed under the total carbohydrate heading because it is partially absorbed as a carbohydrate.

Never subtract sugar alcohol from the total carbohydrate grams when reading a food label. Many companies list a product's net carb grams on its front labeling. The low grams advertised may look temptingly good, but there is a chance that such companies are subtracting both dietary fiber *and* sugar alcohol from the total carbohydrate grams. This is not a legitimate net carb amount because part of the sugar alcohol will affect blood sugar and insulin release. Don't be deceived; read the real ingredient label to get the true picture.

FREE ZONES

Now that you have a sense of the easy carb counting you'll do on Step One, take enjoyment from the fact that you won't have to count a thing in the lean proteins, healthy fat, vegetable, and other "liberal" categories. There is no food weighing, measuring, or counting of "free

BE CAREFUL WITH LOW-CARB RECIPES

The carbohydrate in most "low-carb" recipes exceeds the Step One limit. Even products designed for other low-carb diets will rarely fit Step One of the Miracle. *When in doubt, stay with the recipes in this book that are permitted for Step One.*

foods" during Step One. Have them any time in reasonable quantities and you'll continue to lose weight and feel great.

THE PROTEIN-FAT PACK: MEAT, CHEESE, NUTS, AND MORE

Lean proteins have the green light in the Miracle program, so eat them liberally. Skinless poultry, lean cuts of beef, reduced-fat cheese, egg whites, and other proteins will provide your body with a sense of satisfaction and staying power. While prime rib and sirloin

A DAY IN THE LIFE OF STEP ONE

Debbie began her first day of the Metabolism Miracle excited about the program that would finally match her body's needs but somewhat anxious about cutting out the carbs. She usually began her day heavy in carbohydrates with either cereal, a bran muffin, or a bagel. To start her new regimen, she instead had a breakfast of scrambled eggs and low-carb toast with whipped butter. She sipped her coffee and she thought, "I can do this."

As her breakfast digested, the only item that contributed to her blood glucose was the low-carb toast. Debbie's brain barely sensed this tiny rise in blood sugar (and since the toast contained only 5 grams of carb, her brain didn't call on the pancreas for an insulin release). Within two hours of eating her breakfast, Debbie heard the coffee cake on the counter calling her name.

She remembered my telling her to stay strong and ignore the cravings for the first three days. She grabbed a handful of almonds and went on with her day.

Right before lunch, Debbie got very hungry. She longed for the cold pizza slice in the refrigerator, but she heard me say, "Ignore the cravings, eat anything on the free list, and move on." So, she grabbed a low-carb wrap, filled it with lean roast beef and Lorraine Swiss, lettuce, tomato, and a dab of mayo, and called it lunch. She was filled up and felt, I can do this.

As the afternoon wore on, Debbie got very tired. She yearned for some chocolate and a nap. She realized that this was her brain, trying to get her to give in and take some preferred fuel—carbohydrate. She reassured herself, ate a spoonful of peanut butter and a protein shake, and went on with her day.

Dinner was no problem. Her energy had returned; she was proud of how well she was doing with her program and was thrilled that Step One required are both proteins, only the sirloin, because of its low-fat profile, is on the recommended protein list. Your body will always burn the fat from what you have eaten before it will burn your fat stores. The sirloin will help you take full advantage of your body's new fat-burning mode.

When you choose lean proteins, healthy fats, and vegetables found on the arrow list, you won't have to concern yourself with serving sizes. You can even, on occasion, choose a protein with a higher fat content. Just remember that after day three of your program, your body has transitioned to a fat-burning mode and you want to take full

---

A Day in the Life of Step One (continued)

no special preparation. She sat down with her family to grilled chicken with broccoli, a large salad, and a heaping cup of sugar-free gelatin with light whipped cream for dessert. Life was good.

Things got tough at 9:00 p.m., when Debbie walked into the kitchen. "Mom, can we have popcorn?" "Honey, while you're in there, would you get me some ice cream?"

Debbie muttered under her breath, "Are they crazy? They know I'm watching carbs and they want me to get the carb snacks that they will eat in front of me?" Just when she was about to snap at her family, she remembered, "One step in front of the other for three days and then hunger and cravings will pass." While the popcorn popped and before she dished out the ice cream, she grabbed a Step One Chocolate Brownie Muffin (recipe on page 276) that she had made earlier in the day. As everyone else snacked, so did Debbie.

Later that night, while her family fell asleep and Debbie had time to read and unwind, she had a cup of Cinnamon Ricotta Pudding (see recipe on page 279) and thought, *I can do this.* And she did.

She carried on, maneuvering effortlessly through the next few days and finding it easy knowing exactly which foods were allowed with no need to weigh or measure them. She indulged in occasional carbs by following the 5x5 rule.

Soon, day four arrived. Sure enough, Debbie woke up with a bit more energy, and she couldn't believe that in such a short time, she was accustomed to her program, had eaten a meal in a restaurant with no problem, felt no carb cravings, and had more energy. Debbie continued with Step One for the full eight weeks and looked forward to Step Two.

advantage of that by choosing lean or light proteins so your body won't waste time burning fat from the food. Instead, it will focus on burning your excess fat.

The "Yes" Lists

Choose any of these proteins during *any* step of the Metabolism Miracle:

LEAN PROTEINS

Poultry

Chicken and turkey   Cornish game hen
  (white meat, skinless)

Be sure to eat poultry without the fatty skin. (Rotisseried chicken, turkey bacon, turkey sausage, turkey kielbasa all have a higher fat content, so limit their use.)

Beef

Flank steak	London broil
Sirloin	85–93% ground beef
T-bone steak, trimmed	Tenderloin
Ground round	Rib roast
Porterhouse steak, trimmed	Rump roast
Filet mignon	Chuck roast
Round steak	

Because most people with untreated Metabolism B have elevated cholesterol, they are advised by their physicians or cardiologists to limit red meat. The fact is that lean cuts of red meat are fine to enjoy on a regular basis. USDA Select cuts are leanest, USDA Choice grades have moderate fat, and USDA Prime cuts contain the most fat. In any case, always trim any visible fat.

Fish and Shellfish

Cod

Tuna (fresh or canned in water)

Trout

Snapper

Flounder

Herring (not creamed)

Tilapia

Whiting

Haddock

Sardines

Sea bass

Pollock

Halibut

Swordfish

Mahimahi

Clams

Crab

Oysters

Lobster

Shrimp

Scallops

Imitation shellfish

Eat fish and seafood broiled, grilled, boiled, or steamed as long as you omit any breading, coating, or cocktail sauce.

Pork

Pork tenderloin

Canadian bacon

Canned, cured, or boiled ham

Trimmed pork chops

Fresh ham

Deli ham

Center-cut loin chops

Many cuts of pork are lean, but pork "products" such as sausage and patties contain added fat you should avoid.

Lamb, Veal, and Game

Roast lamb

Lamb chop

Leg of lamb

Lean veal chop

Veal roast

Venison

Skinless duck

Ostrich

Deer

Buffalo

Skinless pheasant

Rabbit

Be sure to trim all visible fat.

Cheese

Low-fat cheese

Low-fat cottage cheese

Grated cheese, such as Parmesan

Cheese with 5 grams or less fat
   per ounce

Part-skim ricotta, mozzarella,
   string cheese

Choose low-fat cheeses and
   cottage cheese with 1% or 2%
   milk fat.

I prefer low-fat cheeses over fat-free choices because the latter tends to be plasticlike and refuses to melt. Nutrition fact labeling lists the serving size for cheese as 1 ounce. If cheese has 5 grams or less fat per ounce, it is a low-fat cheese.

You may choose regular cheese, but be aware that your body will spend time burning the fat from the cheese instead of the fat off your body. Be aware when eating out: Restaurants rarely carry low-fat cheeses, so you may choose to have regular cheese when eating out, but stock your home or office refrigerator with the low-fat variety.

Eggs

Whole eggs (maximum 5   Egg whites
  yolks/week)   Egg substitute

Eat as many egg whites or as much egg substitute as you like, as they contain no fat. Try to limit your egg yolks to five per week. When making an omelet, for example, use two or three egg whites but only one of the yolks.

Soy Products

Tofu   *Vegetarian or soy-based meat
*Unsweetened soy milk   substitutes

A half cup (4 ounces) of tofu has as much high-quality protein as an ounce of meat.

When you opt for vegetarian meat substitutes such as veggie burgers or veggie nuggets, use the net carb rule to be sure that they have 5 grams or less per serving. Some veggie products contain hidden carbohydrate from chickpeas, lentils, or kidney beans.

TAKE OFF YOUR COAT

You may use any cooking method for proteins except those that depend upon coating the meat or fish with flour, bread crumbs, sweetened sauces, gravies, or sweet marinades.

Grilling, baking, roasting, sautéing, and broiling all pass muster with the *Metabolism Miracle* plan. For additional flavoring, use carb-free spices or seasonings, such as mustard, vinegar, and garlic. Citrus and wine can also be used in cooking.

"SWEETENED" PEANUT BUTTER

If you miss the taste of your childhood peanut butters, which were often hydrogenated and sweetened, try making your own from natural versions:

1. Remove the top from the natural peanut butter jar.
2. Microwave for about 30 seconds to soften the peanut butter.
3. Stir in two (1 g) packets of Splenda and, if desired, a pinch of salt.
4. Store in the refrigerator.

Peanut and Nut Butters

Natural peanut butter (refrigerate after opening)

Natural almond butter (refrigerate after opening)

*Processed peanut butter or nut butters (use 5x5 rule)

Natural peanut butter, with only peanuts and optional salt as ingredients, offers the best choice during Step One because most processed peanut butter is sweetened with sugar. Just as you don't have to be concerned about the carb content of nuts, you don't have to count the carb in natural peanut butter. Processed peanut butter will require counting as a 5x5 food, due to added sugar.

*Reduced-Carbohydrate Protein Shakes

These premixed ready-to-drink shakes have the protein of about 3 ounces of meat along with added vitamins and minerals. You can find them in the supermarket or pharmacy. Most have only 1 to 3 grams of net carbohydrate.

---

* Starred items must be checked with the net carb formula and must fit into the 5x5 rule. (See "Easy Carb Counting," page 54.)

HOW MUCH IS TOO MUCH?

Keep in mind that although the majority of your excess weight is due to the overprocessing of carbohydrate, large portion sizes of proteins and fats will also contribute to your weight. If you consume excessive quantities of meats and fats, your body will have no choice but to store the excess as fat.

For that reason, unlike some other low-carb diets, the Metabolism Miracle will never suggest that you eat a quarter-pound of bacon, drench your salad in blue cheese dressing, or smother your broccoli with heaping spoonfuls of butter. But you can have Canadian bacon, balsamic vinaigrette, and broccoli with a touch of whipped butter and continue to lose fat and weight.

I once had a patient who took the words "eat liberally" literally. She ate a jar of natural peanut butter a day. I pointed out that although the natural peanut butter was in the protein arrow and not considered a carb in the Miracle program, it *was* a high-fat item. Peanuts and peanut oil, albeit healthy fats, are still fats. So . . . all the while she had followed Step One and steered her body into the fat-burning mode, she had been sabotaging herself by burning the peanut butter's fat! Use common sense and consume normal portions of lean protein, heart-healthy fat, and low-carb veggies.

HEART-HEALTHY FATS

Butter/Margarine

Whipped butter

Light butter

Butter blends (half butter, half oil)

Light, tub, and whipped margarines (avoid hydrogenation)

For years, butter has had a bad reputation because it is made from the saturated fat of milk. Margarine is made of vegetable oil, which is not a saturated fat. On the surface, oil seems like a healthier alternative to the use of a saturated fat, right? Wrong. The healthy oil used in margarine was made spreadable by pumping in hydrogen (called *hydrogenation*). This process jarred the oil's fat chains and broke them apart, releasing *free radicals*, trans fats that have been linked to certain kinds of cancer. Note the rise in stomach and colon cancer from the advent of margarine, vegetable shortening, creamy peanut butter, and mass-produced baked goods after the late 1940s.

If you are choosing margarine or spread, you must look for a product that contains no trans fats. Check the ingredient list for *no* partial hydrogenation. The first ingredient should be *liquid* oil, not partially hydrogenated oil.

Oils

Olive oil

Canola oil

Peanut oil

Safflower oil

Sunflower oil

Corn oil

Vegetable oil

Salad Dressings

Most regular dressings and true vinaigrettes contain a very small amount of carbohydrate but vinaigrettes contain even less. Use regular salad dressing in a light amount, to keep your fat intake down without added carbohydrate. The age-old technique of taking salad on your fork and dipping it lightly into your salad dressing on the side really does help to cut down on your total fat consumption.

Avoid fat-free salad dressings. The manufacturer generally replaces the flavor of the fat with sugar, making their carb count climb into the danger zone. If you are consuming a lower-fat dressing that contains carb, make sure that the portion you are using is less than 5 grams of carb.

Mayonnaise

Light or low-fat preferred

Olives
Green, black, stuffed

Nuts
Almonds, cashews, pecans, pistachios, and walnuts are all good choices. Also, peanuts, technically legumes, are acceptable. Avoid honey-roasted nuts, however, because honey is a natural sugar coating. If you have a condition called diverticulosis or if you are having stomach or intestinal upset, check with your physician. Some physicians tell these patients to chew nuts into a smooth paste before swallowing, to ease their digestion.

A handful of nuts in the midmorning, midafternoon, and evening can be a great choice of snack. Although they have carbohydrate, the healthy fat content of nuts slows their digestion and the carbohydrate is released so slowly that it is negligible to your blood glucose. Spread your intake of nuts throughout the day and don't go overboard with the quantity. I once had a patient who consumed five pounds of pistachios in one afternoon. She called the office in the late afternoon, complaining of stomach pains!

Sesame Seeds, Pumpkin Seeds, Sunflower Seeds
Tahini paste (ground sesame seeds; use as a dip or a spread for
   vegetables)

Avocado
Avocado has heart-healthy monounsaturated fats, but keep in mind that one avocado has the fat content of 8 teaspoons of oil!

Sour Cream or Cream Cheese
Light or reduced fat is recommended.

Creamer or Half-and-Half

Light or low-fat is recommended. When using *flavored creamers, check against the net carb test and count them as a 5x5 carb. Regular half-and-half, used lightly because of its high fat content, is also fine.

NEUTRAL VEGETABLES

Go to town eating the following vegetables. With the exception of tomatoes and tomato products that must be limited (see "Tomato Tip," page 71), you may eat these vegetables at any time and in any quantity even during Step One. They are filled with vitamins, minerals, fiber, and antioxidants for great health.

Artichoke

Artichoke hearts

Asparagus

Green beans, wax beans

Bean sprouts

Broccoli

Brussels sprouts

Cabbage

Cauliflower

Celery

Cucumber

Dill pickles

Eggplant

Onions and scallions

Greens such as collards, kale,
   mustard, and turnip greens

Kohlrabi

Leeks

Mushrooms

Okra

Peppers (all colors)

Radishes

Salad greens, including all lettuce,
   endive, escarole, romaine

Summer squash or zucchini

Spaghetti squash

Sauerkraut

Spinach

Tomato (maximum 1/meal)

Cherry tomatoes (maximum
   10/meal)

*Tomato juice (4 ounces/meal)

*Vegetable juice (4 ounces/meal)

*Canned tomatoes (1/2
   cup/meal)

Turnips

*Salsa (1/2 cup/meal)

You'll notice that certain vegetables, such as carrots, beets, and peas, don't show up on this list. These vegetables contain enough carbohydrate in the amount that will disrupt Step One. Instead, focus on the many veggies above that will keep your pancreas resting and your fat burning.

TOMATO TIP

Think of tomatoes as a cross between a fruit and a vegetable. Like many fruits, they have a certain amount of carbohydrate and, for that reason, you should limit them during Step One to a half cup per meal.

Most commercial or prepared tomato sauce is not allowed during Step One as it contains added sugar or concentrated paste. Consider making a quick marinara sauce of crushed tomatoes, garlic, onions, wine, and olive oil. A half-cup serving of this sauce is permitted on Step One as a 5x5 carb choice. Use it on steamed vegetables or as a sauce for chicken or fish.

FREEBIES DURING STEP ONE

During Step One, you can have these foods whenever you like, if their carb grams are zero:

Sweet Treats
Sugar-free gelatin
Sugar-free chewing gum   Sugar-Free ice pops
Sugar-free jelly
Sugar-free syrup

Basics
Bouillon   Consommé
Broth

Beverages

Club soda

Diet soda

Sugar-free tonic

Coffee

Tea

Select fitness water, flavored
  waters, and flavored seltzers

Condiments

White horseradish

Lemon and lime juice

Mustard

Dill pickles

Vinegar

Herbs

Spices

THE LOW-CARB, LOW-SUGAR BANDIT

One brand of ice pop features the Splenda logo. The label states, "Use in low-carb diets," and on the front is declared: "4 grams of net carb!" The pops seem perfect for Step One, right? Look again, this time with the net carb formula to help you:

Serving Size: 1 ice pop
Total Carbohydrate: 12 grams
Dietary Fiber: 4 grams
Sugar: 4 grams
Sugar Alcohol: 4 grams

12 grams (total carb) − 4 grams (dietary fiber) = **8 grams (net carbs)**

Because the pops contain sugar alcohol as well as sugar, the real answer for net carb is not the 4 grams promoted on the front of the package, but 8 grams! This product is not allowed on Step One of your diet.

Companies get away with faulty math because the FDA currently has no set formula for net carb. The ice pop manufacturer subtracted both the dietary fiber **and** the sugar alcohol grams to come up with 4 net carbs listed on the front of the package. But sugar alcohol affects blood glucose and if you inadvertently slipped this food into your diet on Step One, your pancreas would release insulin and set you back.

Most low-carb products on your store's shelves similarly misrepresent the net carb grams on the front of their packages. *Always* use the net carb formula to protect yourself.

WHAT ABOUT ALCOHOLIC BEVERAGES?

In their unfermented form, grapes and grains pack quite a few carbs. But once fermented or distilled, they chemically change into alcohol that no longer follows the body's carbohydrate pathway. As a result, alcohol does not cause blood glucose to spike in the way carbohydrate would.

During Step One, your liver, the organ that helps to clean alcohol from the bloodstream, is on temporary vacation. While it rests, it may

THE BUZZ ON BEER

Regular beer is not allowed on the Miracle program because it contains too much carbohydrate, even after fermentation. Light beer, on the other hand, is processed further and the result is often diluted with water, bringing its carb content into the acceptable range.

be a bit slower to process alcohol and as a result you will feel alcohol's effects faster and for a longer time. So although one or two drinks in a night will probably fit into Step One of the Metabolism Miracle, please drink alcohol wisely and slowly to feel its effect before continuing.

Be sure to consult your physician regarding alcohol because certain medications and health conditions such as diabetes can change your reaction to alcohol. On the Metabolism Miracle program, the maximum recommended amount of alcohol (and only with physician approval) is one or two alcohol-containing beverages. A "drink" is defined as:

5 ounces wine

12 ounces light beer

1 1/2 ounces spirits (gin, vodka, whiskey)

STEP ONE SAMPLE MENUS

DAY 1

Breakfast

Egg substitute omelet with chopped peppers, onions, and tomato

1 slice low-carb toast (5 g net carb) with whipped butter and sugar-
    free jelly

Coffee with half-and-half and Splenda

Midmorning Snack

Handful of almonds and 1 string cheese

16 ounces flavored water

Lunch

1 low-carb wrap (4 g net carb) filled with sliced turkey breast, sliced
   cheese, shredded lettuce, tomato, and mayonnaise
Sugar-free gelatin
16 ounces water with lemon

Afternoon Snack

Strawberry protein shake (1 g net carb)
Celery sticks with peanut butter

Dinner

Lean grilled burger
Generous piece of Pasta-Free Veggie Lasagne (recipe on page 264)
Tossed salad with balsamic vinaigrette
Lemon Ricotta Pudding (recipe on page 281)
16 ounces decaffeinated green tea

Nighttime Snacks

Handful of nuts, string cheese, Chocolate Brownie Muffin (recipe on
   page 276) (5 g net carb)

DAY 2

Breakfast

Vanilla protein shake (1 g net carb)
Handful of almonds

Midmorning Snack

Spoonful of natural peanut butter with celery sticks
Decaffeinated coffee with half-and-half and Splenda

Lunch (ordered from Chinese take-out)
Egg drop soup
Steamed shrimp and vegetables with no sauce (use some of the egg
    drop soup as your "sauce")
Green tea

Afternoon Snack
String cheese and handful of almonds
16 ounces water

Dinner
Grilled chicken Caesar salad (no croutons) with dressing on the side
Low-carb tortilla (5 g net carb)
Sugar-free gelatin with light whipped cream
16 ounces flavored water

Nighttime Snacks
Chocolate Ricotta Pudding (recipe on page 280)
Handful of Parmesan Chips (recipe on page 236)

BREAKFAST IDEAS FOR STEP ONE

Egg white omelet with peppers, onions, tomato, and mushrooms, or
    egg white or egg substitute omelet with ham and low-fat Cheddar
1 slice low-carb toast (5 g or less net carb) with whipped butter

4 ounces vegetable juice (5 g or less net carb)
Scoop of low-fat cottage cheese or part-skim ricotta cheese sprinkled
    with walnuts and cinnamon

Low-carb chocolate shake (5 g or less net carb)
Handful of peanuts

Easy Egg Cups (recipe on page 225)
1 slice Canadian bacon
1 slice low-carb toast (5 g or less net carb)

Low-carb yogurt smoothie (5 g or less net carb)
Handful of almonds

1 slice low-carb bread (5 g or less net carb) with melted cheese and
    tomato slices

Low-carb tortilla wrap (5 g or less net carb) spread with natural peanut
    butter

Low-carb yogurt (5 g or less net carb)
Celery sticks with peanut butter

1 slice low-carb bread (5 g or less net carb) spread with low-fat cream
    cheese and sugar-free jelly

Miracle Quiche (recipe page 226)
Zucchini Muffin (5 g or less net carb) (recipe page 278)

6 Silver Dollar Pancakes (recipe on page 229) with whipped butter
    and sugar-free syrup
2 strips turkey bacon

1 slice low-carb toast (5 g or less carb) with 1 tablespoon of natural
    peanut butter
1 cup unsweetened soy milk

1 slice low-carb toast (5 g or less carb) spread with low-fat ricotta
    cheese and cinnamon; heat in a toaster oven until warm

LUNCH IDEAS FOR STEP ONE

Tuna salad with light mayonnaise on a bed of crisp lettuce and
    tomato wedges
Sugar-free gelatin

Egg Drop Soup
Chicken Caesar salad without croutons and with Caesar dressing on
    the side (use sparingly)

Chef's salad with ham, cheese, egg, turkey, and low-fat cheese, with
    light dressing on the side
Parmesan Chips (recipe on page 236)

Sirloin burger without the bun, with low-carb ketchup and lettuce,
    tomato, and onion as desired
Side salad with light dressing

Miracle Grilled Cheese (recipe on page 234)
Tomato wedges
Cinnamon Ricotta Pudding (recipe on page 279)

Turkey and light cheese roll-ups with peppers and tomatoes, wrapped
    in a low-carb tortilla wrap (5 g or less net carb)
Sugar-free gelatin

Low-carb yogurt (5 g or less net carb)
Ham and cheese roll-ups
Celery sticks with peanut butter

Light cottage cheese in a hollowed red bell pepper "cup"
Tossed salad with balsamic vinaigrette
1 slice low-carb toast spread with garlic butter (5 g or less net carb)

Grilled chicken strips over romaine lettuce leaves sprinkled with feta
    cheese and almonds
Light dressing

Italian Vegetable Soup (recipe on page 244)
Turkey/cheese roll-ups
Handful of Parmesan Chips (recipe on page 236)

Shrimp salad with light mayonnaise over a bed of dark greens
Lemon Ricotta Pudding (recipe on page 281)

Chunky Chicken Salad (recipe on page 254) and sun-dried tomatoes
    on a crisp salad base, with low-fat dressing of choice

1 slice low-carb bread (5 g or less net carb) with natural peanut butter
    and sugar-free jelly
Celery sticks with cream cheese
Sugar-free gelatin with whipped topping

Easy Pizza (recipe on page 232)
Antipasti: ham, fresh mozzarella, black olives, and tomatoes

DINNER IDEAS FOR STEP ONE

Roasted chicken breast with fat-free gravy (5 g or less net carb)
Mashed Cauliflower (recipe on page 270)
Green beans amandine

London broil steak with sautéed mushrooms
1 slice low-carb garlic toast (5 g or less net carb)
Tossed salad with light dressing
Broccoli with light cheese sauce

Broiled flounder
Oven-roasted peppers, onions, and zucchini
Mashed Cauliflower (recipe on page 270)
Sugar-free gelatin with whipped topping

Miracle "Spaghetti" (recipe on page 255)
1 slice low-carb garlic bread (5 g or less net carb)
Caesar salad with light dressing

Chicken Paprikash (recipe on page 253)
Steamed green beans
Chocolate Brownie Muffin (recipe on page 276 with light whipped
    cream topping

Chicken broth with "free" veggies
Tender Spinach Salad (recipe on page 246)
Handful of Parmesan Chips (recipe on page 236)
Sugar-free ice pop

Sliced turkey breast with low-fat gravy
Broccoli-Cheese Casserole (recipe on page 269)
"Guilded" Cinnamon Muffin (recipe on page 277)

Pork tenderloin
Roasted vegetables
Tossed salad with light dressing
No-sugar-added pudding (5 g or less net carb)

Sirloin burger on a grilled portobello mushroom (as a bun), with low-fat cheese, low-carb ketchup, and lettuce, tomato, and onion
Raw vegetables (no carrots) with low-fat onion dip

Broiled tilapia
Broiled tomatoes with Parmesan cheese
Steamed spinach
Sugar-free gelatin with whipped topping

Turkey hot dogs with mustard in a low-carb wrap (5 g or less net carb)
Sweet-and-Sour Cukes (recipe on page 245)
Sugar-free ice pop

Veggie or meatless burger (5 g or less net carb) and light cheese, open faced on 1 slice of low-carb bread (5 g or less net carb) with low-carb ketchup
Cabbage Salad (recipe on page 241)

Grilled Pork Chop
Mashed Cauliflower (recipe on page 270)
Broccoli crowns
Side salad with light dressing
Sugar-free gelatin with whipped topping

Baked chicken breast
Sweet-and-Sour Cukes (recipe on page 245)
Roasted eggplant and peppers
Square of dark chocolate (5 g or less net carb)

SNACK IDEAS FOR STEP ONE

Many people choose to use noncarb snacks and save their 5x5 carb choices for mealtime and bedtime. Remember not to stack carbs during Step One—you have the option to choose up to 5 grams of net carb in no briefer than a five-hour period.

Part-skim string cheese
Light-cheese wedges
Low-fat cottage cheese
Nuts
Spoonful of natural peanut butter
Celery sticks with natural peanut butter or light cream cheese
Veggies with light dip
Olives
Turkey or ham and cheese rolls
Low-carb shake (5 g or less net carb)
Protein shake (5 g or less net carb)
Low-carb yogurt or smoothie (5 g or less net carb)
Low-carb or sugar-free hot chocolate (5 g or less net carb)
Sugar-free ice pop
Sugar-free gelatin with whipped topping
Parmesan Chips (recipe on page 236)
Parmesan Chips (recipe on page 236) with salsa (5 g or less net carb)
Meringue cookies (5 g or less net carb)
Ricotta Puddings (recipes on pages 279–281) (5 g or less net carb)
Crispy Tortilla Chips (recipe on page 235) (5 g or less net carb)
Chocolate Brownie Muffin (recipe on page 276) (5 g or less net carb)
"Guilded" Cinnamon Muffin (recipe on page 277) (5 g or less carb)
Zucchini Muffin (recipe on page 278) (5 g or less net carb)

STEP ONE—FREQUENTLY ASKED QUESTIONS

I got on the scale after seven days on Step One and saw no weight loss. What's going on?

When you begin the Metabolism Miracle, take your starting weight and body measurements (see chapter 10) and don't step back on that scale for at least a full month. Remember, this program not only brings about permanent weight loss but also cleans up excesses in fats and sugar, and rests your pancreas and liver. Only after the third day when your liver has emptied its glycogen stores will you begin burning excess fat; seven days is too soon to see a change in weight.

Follow the plan, get physically active, take one day at a time, and measure your progress in eight weeks. The results will be worth the wait!

For the past eight weeks, everyone has remarked that I look great. I feel rested and energized and I've tightened my belt three holes. Why does it look like I've lost twice as much as the scale says?

On every other diet plan, you lose a combination of water, fat, and muscle. Steps One and Two of the Metabolism Miracle are fat-burning phases. Fat is light, fluffy, big-volume tissue. When you lose ten pounds of fat, it looks and feels like twenty.

The Miracle leaves what your body needs—muscle and water—and burns excess fat. Your clothes will fit as if you've lost twice the amount; and your lipids, blood pressure, and blood sugar will improve as if you've lost double the scale weight. Celebrate your loss and look forward to more!

Two weeks into Step One, I caved and ate a brownie! What now?

Get back on track right now. The longer you wait, the harder it will be to restart. Continue to count the two weeks you put into the program and begin your next six weeks on Step One. If you really fell out of line, with three or more indiscretions in one week, it would be best to go back to the beginning of your eight-week program.

I'm constipated during Step One. Help!

You probably aren't drinking the 64 ounces of caffeine-free fluid you need each day. In Steps One and Two, fat-burning phases, your kidneys will cleanse your bloodstream of the breakdown products of fat-burning, and your body will flush this waste out with urine. If you don't drink adequate fluid, your body will take needed fluid from your tissues and even your gastrointestinal tract, and you will be left with hardened, difficult-to-pass stools. Even if you aren't thirsty drink, drink, drink!

Also be sure to keep up your fiber intake with raw vegetables, salads, nuts, and 5x5 whole-grain bread products. Two teaspoons of a fiber supplement powder, made of powdered plant fiber, can add 10 grams of fiber with no extra carb. Finally, exercise is critical to keep things moving along.

I found a pudding marked "Sugar-Free/Use on a Low-Carb Diet." How do I know if it's okay to eat during Step One?

There is only one way to determine if a food is right for Step One. Check the nutrition facts label and do the net carb formula: Total carb grams – dietary fiber grams = net carbs.

If a serving's net carb is less than or equal to 5 grams, it is suitable for Step One.

How many 5-gram net carb foods can I have at a meal?

Use the 5x5 rule: Limit yourself to 5 grams of net carb in a five-hour period. I usually suggest that you spread apart your 5 gram net carbs among breakfast, lunch, dinner, and bedtime. When you place them closer, in midmorning or late afternoon snacks, you risk stacking them and breaking the 5x5 rule.

Remember that you don't have to count carbs for most of the lean protein, vegetable, or health fat choices (page 49). Only questionable foods (or those marked *) must be checked.

I have type 2 diabetes, take oral medication, and maintain a blood sugar of 200 mg/dL (11.1 mmol/L). Two weeks into Step One I find myself feeling a little shaky, dizzy, and sweaty but when I check my blood sugar, it's normal—for the first time in years. Why am I feeling as if it's going too low?

Anyone with diabetes who takes medication to lower blood sugar (either oral or insulin) should inform his or her physician before beginning this program. Step One quickly improves blood sugar. Because your blood sugar has been out of control for a while, your brain has come to accept that 200 mg/dL as a normal reading, so the new "normal" level strikes your body as too low and you get all the symptoms of low blood sugar. As long as your blood sugar is in the normal range (over 70 mg/dL [3.9 mmol/L]), you do not need to treat it. Sit down, sip some water, relax, and the feeling will pass.

If you do not take medication for diabetes (oral medication or insulin), you will not become hypoglycemic on this program. If you are taking medication to reduce blood sugar and your blood sugar dips beneath 70 mg/dL (3.9 mmol/L), you have true hypoglycemia and must immediately treat the condition. Be sure to report low blood sugar readings ASAP to your doctor so that he or she may decrease the dosage of your medication and you can continue right along with Step One at a lesser medication dosage.

Can I eat as much as I want of the allowed foods on Step One?

Normal portion sizes of these foods are fine. For example, if you are hungry, there's no problem with having 8 ounces of lean protein at a meal. Huge portions, however, will thwart your weight loss. If you are hungry at any time, you can eat! Just make sure that the foods you choose are from the approved foods list, and consumed in reasonable portions.

STEP TWO—TRANSITION: A HEALTHY PATH TO CARBS

STEP TWO BASICS

Time: 8 weeks or longer, until you reach your desired weight
Challenge: Reintroduce healthy carbohydrates in the proper amount and at the right time, to promote continued fat burning and weight loss. Gently restart your rested pancreas and liver.
Result: Steady weight loss and continued improvements in blood sugar, cholesterol, triglycerides, blood pressure, and energy

During the eight weeks of Step One, you have lost fat inches and unwanted pounds. You no longer crave carbs and you feel more energized than you have in years. You have completed your spring cleaning.

While you can feel and see the benefits of Step One, it helps to understand what internal changes have occurred to retune your metabolism. Your overactive pancreas has rested and your liver has significantly decreased releasing glycogen. Your blood lipids (cholesterol and triglycerides) have markedly improved. Your fat cells have begun to shrink and your insulin keys better fit the receptors on your

BEFORE AND AFTER

Measure your progress in Steps Two and Three by stepping on the scale and taking your body measurements (chapter 10) only once a month. That way, you'll see dramatic changes without the erratic ups and downs of daily weight fluctuations.

cells. In short, your Metabolism B has been put in order so that it can behave normally. Step Two helps to reprogram it to process carbohydrates normally.

Now you are ready to reintroduce carbohydrates, the fuel that a healthy body needs to run properly. To do that, you must learn three key skills:

1. How to introduce the mildest carbohydrates to a pancreas that has been resting for eight weeks
2. How to choose the right amount of carbohydrate at meals and snacks for continued weight loss and fat burn
3. How to place carbohydrate throughout the day. Timing is everything!

All of the foods that you ate freely in Step One, you will continue to eat as base foods for Step Two. In addition, you will now add carb servings from a long list of low-impact carb foods. These foods will allow your pancreas to wake up slowly, preventing it from overreacting with excess insulin.

Step Two is a nutritionally balanced diet that allows safe, long-term weight loss. Plan to stay in this part of the program for at least eight weeks, until you have reached your desired weight. There is no limit to the amount of time you may stay on Step Two.

"But I'm Happy with Step One, and I Don't Want to Move On!"

After eight weeks on Step One, many patients tell me, "I never want to eat carbohydrate foods again. I look great, feel great, and my lab work is great. Why should I eat the food that caused all my problems?"

The cause of their problems was not carbohydrate. The cause stemmed from their Metabolism B overreacting to carbohydrate. Now that their system is back in balance, if they reintroduce carbohydrate the proper way, they will continue to lose weight and feel great.

My patients' carbohydrate phobia comes from their past experiences with other low-carb diets. When these programs reintroduce carbohydrate to the diet, low-impact carbohydrate is rarely emphasized. These diets offer no guidance on how much carbohydrate to introduce to the rested metabolism and when to schedule it into the day. Without proper guidelines regarding the introduction of carb, people with Metabolism B head right back to square one and experience rapid weight gain, low energy, and declining health.

As invigorating as Step One has proven for you, it is not healthy or normal to live on a very low-carb diet for longer than eight weeks at a time. **Very** low-carb phases are not nutritionally balanced and eating this way for long periods of time will leave your pancreas and liver languid. Like every organ of the body, these two are designed to function. If they rest for too long, they may not perform efficiently when called upon in the future.

The Metabolism Miracle, in contrast to other low-carb diets, gives you very clear instructions on how to do reintroduce carbohydrates the healthy way, continue to lose weight, and rediscover the joy in eating the many carbohydrate choices that fit this program.

How It Works

Let's take a look inside your body to understand exactly what happens when you reintroduce carbohydrates on Step Two.

For the past eight weeks on Step One, your liver was intentionally depleted of glycogen stores so that it could not engage and cause blood sugar to rise and prod the pancreas into overreleasing insulin. Instead, both organs have rested. On the morning that you begin Step Two, the correct amount of low-impact carbohydrate will gently enter your bloodstream and glycogen will once again be stored in the liver.

Once the liver has filled with glycogen, it is poised and ready to do its job. When you delay or skip a meal or fast during nighttime sleep, the liver goes into survival mode and releases a meal's worth of glycogen into your bloodstream. Every time your liver feeds you in this way, your pancreas overreleases the fat-gain hormone, insulin. The more often it happens, the more frazzled the pancreas becomes. Before you know it, your pancreas returns to overreleasing insulin, fat cells expand, insulin keys no longer fit the receptors, and hormonal imbalance returns.

Step Two is designed specifically to prevent the above scenario from occurring. By introducing a very specific amount of carbohydrate (11 to 20 grams) no further than five hours apart, the liver will rarely be called upon to release glycogen. This proper reintroduction of carbohydrate minimizes the number of times per day that your liver engages. Consuming the correct amount of carb will also prevent the pancreas from overreacting to blood sugar rises from excess carbohydrate intake. You will take control of your blood sugar and prevent the pancreas from overreacting.

BACK TO THE TRUSTY FORMULA

So how do you keep your carbohydrates within the 11–20 gram range? You already know how to use the net carb formula because of the 5x5 rule in Step One.

Total carbohydrate grams – dietary fiber grams = net carb grams

In Step Two, you'll use the formula to guarantee that foods such as bread, crackers, cereal, bars, yogurt and sugar-free ice cream stay within the 11–20 gram window. For example, you may want to eat a slice of whole-grain toast at breakfast. Whole-grain bread is mentioned on the Step Two "Low-Impact Carbs" list (page 96), but you'll want to make sure that the bread fits into the 11–20 gram allotment. Check the nutrition facts label and plug the numbers into your trusty formula.

Serving Size: 1 Slice
Total Carbohydrate: 20 grams
Dietary Fiber: 3 grams

20 – 3 = **17 net carb grams**

This bread fits into the 11–20 gram window, so go ahead and enjoy it.

At lunch, you decide to have some multigrain crackers with your chicken Caesar salad. How many crackers can you have and still be within the 11–20 gram target range? Simply check the nutrition facts label.

Serving Size: 8 crackers
Total Carbohydrate: 24 grams
Dietary Fiber: 5 grams

24 – 5 = **19 net carb grams**

Eight crackers fit into the 11–20 gram window, so go ahead and enjoy them.

For the next eight weeks, you should choose all of your carb servings from the "Low-Impact Carbs" list (page 96). The whole-grain bread and multigrain crackers are on the list. High-impact carbs such as marshmallows, potato chips, and fruit juice are not on the list. Keep them out of Step Two to prevent yourself from backsliding.

TIMING IS EVERYTHING

Once you enter Step Two, you must not exceed five hours without the inclusion of an 11–20 gram net carb food within every five-hour period, to keep your metabolism stoked, or else your liver will overcompensate with glycogen, you will stress the pancreas, and weight will come back. You'll have created the same metabolic monster that you transformed so successfully in Step One.

Remember that you are reprogramming your body. You want to program it with the right amount of low-impact carb at the right time. This is a period of transition. If you skip the transition and introduce carbs haphazardly, you will most definitely regain everything you've lost.

To recap: During Step Two, you must eat a food from the 11–20 gram net carb list at the following times:

- Prior to exercising if you exercise before breakfast
- With breakfast, lunch, and dinner
- At snacks between meals that are eaten more than five hours apart
- Right before you go to bed at night
- If you wake up during the middle of the night (an 11–20 gram snack is recommended but not required)

You have the option of having two "free" 5x5 carbs daily without adding their carb grams to your 11–20 carb "dam."

Choose all your 11–20 carb servings from the Low-Impact Carbs list (page 96).

What's Magical about 11 to 20 Carb Grams?

Once your liver is back from its vacation, the only way to control blood sugar response involves the timing and the amount of low-impact carb throughout your day.

Time your carbohydrates in the correct portions throughout the day, and you have effectively set up a dam that prevents the liver from releasing glycogen. It is critical to keep the amount of carbohydrate between 11 and 20 grams. A dam built of less than 11 grams will not be high enough to prevent liver glycogen from flowing over. A dam built of more than 20 grams of carbohydrate at a meal or snack will stimulate the pancreas to release extra insulin, and that will lead to weight gain rather than weight loss.

The easiest way to remember the details of Step Two is: Always place *a carb dam (11–20 grams low-impact carb) to block the liver at*:

Breakfast—within one hour of waking up
Lunch
Dinner
Bedtime Snack—as close to bedtime as possible

If the time between breakfast and lunch will exceed five hours, you need to set a reinforcing dam with a midmorning snack (an additional 11–20 carb grams) to keep the liver on hold until you eat lunch. Similarly, if the time between lunch and dinner exceeds five hours, you will set a reinforcing dam with a midafternoon snack (an additional 11–20 grams) to stop the liver from spilling in the fifth hour.

On those days when you need to take the additional 11–20 grams as a between-meal snack, remember to also consume your 11–20 gram carb dam at the next meal. The 11–20 gram carb replacement at breakfast, lunch, dinner, and bedtime is a constant.

These 11 to 20 grams of low-impact carb, placed correctly, is what Step Two is all about. Proper placement enables the pancreas and liver to awaken gently and keep you in a weight-loss mode.

KEEP THEM COMING

It's hard to believe but, once you introduce carbs, you must keep them coming or you will regain weight. It is very possible that you'll need six or more carb servings per day.

Here's a typical day's carb placement for Step Two:

7:00 a.m. — Wake up
8:00 a.m. — Breakfast (11–20 g net carb)
11:00 a.m. — Midmorning Snack with 11–20 g net carb (breakfast and lunch are greater than five hours apart)
1:30 p.m. — Lunch (11–20 g net carb)
4:30 p.m. — Midafternoon Snack with 11–20 g net carb (lunch and dinner are greater than five hours apart)
7:30 p.m. — Dinner (11–20 g net carb)
10:30 p.m. — Bedtime Snack (11–20 g net carb)
11:00 p.m. — Bedtime

(For specific examples, see "Step Two Sample Menu" on page 102.)

THE FIRST THREE DAYS OF STEP TWO

Most people notice that they feel a little bloated and their belts are a tad snugger during the first three days of Step Two. You are **not** gaining weight. As the liver refills with glycogen, it also takes in some additional fluid. Drink plenty of fluid during these days, to help your body release the excess fluid. By the fourth day, the bloating will have disappeared and your waistband will be back to normal.

After those first three days, your body should continue to feel healthy and energized while you continue to lose weight. Learn Step

Two as if it were your job. It will put you in control of your weight and health for life.

As with all of the steps of the Metabolism Miracle, be sure to follow the ten "Rules to Thrive By (chapter 8). Pay particular attention to drinking at least 64 ounces of caffeine-free fluid daily, exercising **a minimum of** thirty minutes, five times a week, and taking the recommended supplements.

Step Two is a nutritionally balanced, safe diet that you can follow for as long as you like and continue to lose weight. Once you have reached the weight that you desire and achieve maximum health on as little medication as possible, step on the scale and check your weight. The weight that makes you healthy and makes you look and feel great is *your* ideal body weight.

Low-Impact Carbs

Choose any food from the low-impact carbs list for your breakfast, lunch, dinner, and bedtime snack. If the time between meals exceeds five hours, place an extra carb serving between them.

All portions shown are "ready to eat" and equal 11–20 grams net carb.

5x5 Carbs

In addition to your necessary 11–20 gram net carb "dams," you may eat two 5x5 carbs on any day during Step Two (see "5x5 Carbs," page 56 .) You needn't add these carbs to the 11–20 gram total. Simply enjoy them as "free carbs."

CEREAL FOR BREAKFAST?

When you want to eat cold cereal and milk for breakfast, remember that the combined milk and cereal net carbs must be 11–20 grams. A half cup of milk has 6 grams of net carb. Choose an unsweetened soy milk or low-carb milk as a free 5x5 carb, and you can have a larger portion of cereal.
Example:

3/4 cup cereal = **9** g net carb
1/2 cup milk = **6** *g net carb*
Total: **15** g net carb

OR

1 1/2 cups cereal = **18** g net carb
1 cup soy or low-carb milk = *"free"* 5x5 *carb*
Total: 18 grams total net carb (you can eat twice the amount of cereal!)

BREADS

Read the label for bread, cereal, "bars" and crackers to make certain that dietary fiber is 2 grams or greater.

2 slices thin-sliced, light, or lower-carb whole-grain bread (2 g fiber or more)
1 slice whole-grain bread (2 g fiber or more)
1 light whole-grain English muffin (2 g fiber or more)
1/2 whole-grain English muffin (2 g fiber or more)
1 light or lower-carb whole-grain pita (2 g fiber or more)
1/2 whole-grain pita (2 g fiber or more)

CEREALS AND GRAINS

1/2 cup cooked oatmeal
1/2 cup cooked barley

BREAD TIPS

FIBER

When you buy breads, crackers, and cereals, make sure they have 2 grams or more of fiber but don't trust the front packaging for that information. Always rely on the nutrition facts label. Grains that contain high amounts of dietary fiber take longer to digest and slow the glucose release into the bloodstream, making them perfect for people with Metabolism B.

Whole wheat bread generally has 2–3 grams of fiber per slice, a perfect choice for Step Two. In contrast, white bread, saltines, cornflakes, and many cereal bars have less than 1 gram of dietary fiber. They will cause blood sugar to spike and your pancreas to overreact.

SPECIALTY BREADS

Give thin-sliced, light, and lower-carb breads a try. With half the carbs of regular breads, they often allow you to have twice as much in your 11–20 net carb allotment.

1 slice of whole wheat bread = 2 slices of light whole wheat bread

Both of these bread choices have 2 grams of fiber or more and between 11 and 20 grams of net carb, making both choices perfect for Step Two.

1/2 cup cooked brown or wild rice
1/2 cup cooked whole-grain pasta (cook al dente)
1/2 cup cooked bulgur
1 serving dry cereal (2 g fiber or more)

CRACKERS AND STARCHY SNACKS

1 serving whole-grain crackers (11–20 g net carb and 2 g or more fiber)
3 cups popcorn (light or hot air–popped without partially hydrogenated oils)

1 serving whole-grain pretzels (11–20 g net carb and 2 g fiber or more)
1 serving tortilla chips (11–20 g net carb and 2 g fiber or more)

PROTEIN BARS

Must contain 11–20 grams of net carb and have 2 g fiber or more.

VEGETABLES AND LEGUMES

1/2 cup corn or 1/2 ear fresh corn
1/2 cup peas
*1/2 cup legumes such as kidney beans, lentils, lima beans, chickpeas,
    white beans, black beans, or white kidney beans*
1/2 whole or 1/2 cup mashed sweet potato or yam
1 cup raw or 1/2 cup cooked carrots
1/2 cup beets

SOUPS

1 cup tomato soup (water-based)
1/2 cup lentil soup
1/2 cup split pea soup

FRUIT

All portions represent 11–20 g net carb. Fruit choices should be average
in size.

1 apple   *1 nectarine*
1 pear   *12 cherries*
1 peach   *1/2 cup natural applesauce*
2 plums

1/2 grapefruit (**avoid** if you are taking the medication Lipitor)

1 cup whole strawberries (6–8 average-size berries)

3/4 cup blackberries

3/4 cup blueberries

1 cup raspberries

2 clementine oranges or 2 small tangerines

8 dried apricot halves

12 grapes

1 orange

3/4 cup pineapple cubes

1/2 banana

FRUIT TIPS

BEWARE OF GIANT FRUIT

When you choose fruit, take stock of its size. You needn't buy the smallest apple in the basket, but the orange that looks more like a basketball isn't a good option, either. Train your eye to focus on average-size fresh fruit that fits into the 11–20 gram net carb rule.

JUST SAY "NO" TO JUICE

With its high-impact carbohydrate and negligible fiber, fruit juice spikes your blood sugar like a rocket, causing the pancreas of anyone with Metabolism B to overreact. Fruit juice is never a good choice if you have Metabolism B.

MISSING YOUR FAVORITE FRUIT?

If a preferred fruit is absent from the Step Two fruit category, it isn't an oversight. The fruits on this list are low impact and fit well into this transition stage when you are being cautious with your pancreas. Other fruits will come back into the picture when you enter Step Three.

MILK AND OTHER DAIRY

1 cup (8 fluid ounces) milk (fat-free, nonfat, 1%, 2%, skim plus)

Plain yogurt (11–20 g net carb)

1 cup (8 fluid ounces) buttermilk (11–20 g net carb)

Fruit-flavored yogurt sweetened with Splenda or sucralose (11–20 g net carb)

1/2 cup sugar-free/fat-free pudding (11–20 g net carb)

No-sugar-added ice cream products sweetened with Splenda (11–20 g net carb)

DAIRY TIPS

HOW LOW CAN YOUR MILK GO?

Eight ounces of milk contain 11–20 grams of net carb, regardless of the milk's fat content. The benefit to using lower-fat versions is that they can help in a fat-burning weight-loss program.

YOGURT CHOICES

An 11–20 gram net carb light yogurt makes a great bedtime snack to keep your liver on hold and your pancreas in check. Don't confuse this light yogurt with the 5x5 version you had in Step One. Five grams of net carb is fine for an anytime snack, but it is not enough carb to "dam" your liver for the night ahead.

WELCOME BACK, ICE CREAM!

Look for ice creams that have sucralose (brand name: Splenda) rather than sugar as the primary sweetener. Even if the net carb appears the same in sugar-sweetened ice cream, the type of carbohydrate is very different from that in Splenda-sweetened products. Sugar-sweetened desserts digest quickly with a high impact that spikes blood glucose.

STEP TWO SAMPLE MENU 1

Remember, timing is critical. You should never go more than five hours without an 11–20 gram net carb serving. In the sample menu below, each 11–20 gram net carb serving is noted, along with two "free" 5x5 carb servings.

6:30 a.m. — *Wake up*

7:00 a.m. — *Breakfast*

> 1 1/2 cups cold cereal (11–20 g net carb) with 8 ounces low-carb milk (3 g carb, a "free" 5x5 carb)
>
> Coffee with half-and-half and Splenda

10:00 a.m. — *Midmorning Snack*

> Handful of peanuts
>
> *You don't need an 11–20 g net carb "dam" because breakfast and lunch are within five hours.*

12:00 noon — *Lunch*

> Grilled cheese sandwich made with 2 slices light whole-grain bread (11–20 g net carb)
>
> Tomato wedges
>
> Iced green tea

4:00 p.m. — *Midafternoon Snack*

> Dip of cottage cheese with 7 sliced strawberries (11–20 g net carb)

6:00 p.m. — *Dinner*

> Broiled flounder
>
> 1/2 cup wild rice (11–20 g net carb)
>
> Steamed broccoli
>
> 1 "Guilded" Cinnamon Muffin (recipe on page 277) (4 g net carb, second "free" 5x5 carb)

10:30 p.m. — *Bedtime Snack*

> 1 serving peach-flavored light yogurt (11–20 g net carb)

Step Two Sample Menu 2

6:00 a.m.—*Preexercise Snack*

    1/2 banana (11–20 g carb)

8:30 *a.m.* —*Breakfast*

    4 ounces tomato juice (4 g net carb, first "free" 5x5 carb)

    Egg substitute with 2 strips turkey bacon

    1 light multigrain English muffin (11–20 g carb) with whipped
        butter

    Coffee

    Because breakfast and lunch are within five hours, you won't need a
        midmorning snack.

1:00 *p.m.*—*Lunch*

    Scoop of tuna salad on a bed of romaine lettuce

    15 thin wheat crackers (11–20 g net carb)

    Flavored water

4:00 *p.m.*—*Midafternoon Snack*

    Part-skim string cheese and a handful of cashews

6:00 *p.m.*—*Dinner*

    Roasted turkey breast with fat-free gravy

    1/2 sweet potato (11–20 g net carb)

    Green beans

    Low-carb chocolate pudding (3 g net carb, second "free" 5x5 carb)

    Sparkling water

11:00 *p.m.*—*Bedtime Snack*

    One ice-cream bar, sweetened with sucralose (11–20 g net carb)

Step Two Sample Menus

BREAKFAST SUGGESTIONS FOR STEP TWO

Miracle Quiche (recipe on page 226)
1 light multigrain English muffin (11–20 g net carb) with natural
    peanut butter and sugar-free jelly
Coffee, decaf, or tea with low-fat half-and-half and Splenda

Egg whites or egg substitute with ham and cheese
2 slices light whole-grain toast (11–20 g net carb) spread with
    whipped cream cheese
Coffee, decaf, or tea with low-fat half-and-half and Splenda

Grilled cheese: 2 slices light multigrain bread (11–20 g net carb), low-
    fat Cheddar cheese, tomato slices, and whipped butter
Coffee, decaf, or tea with low-fat half-and-half and Splenda

3/4 cup cereal with 1/2 cup milk (11–20 g net carb)
Coffee, decaf, or tea with low-fat half-and-half and Splenda

1 1/2 cups cereal with carb-controlled milk (11–20 g net carb)
Coffee, decaf, or tea with low-fat half-and-half and Splenda

1/2 cup cooked oatmeal or 1 prepared envelope unflavored cooked
    oatmeal (11–20 g net carb)
Sprinkle of cinnamon, walnuts, and Splenda
Coffee, decaf, or tea with low-fat half-and-half and Splenda

2 slices thin-sliced whole-grain toast (11–20 g net carb) spread with 1
    teaspoon sugar-free jelly and 1 tablespoon natural peanut butter

1 cup carb-controlled milk (5x5 carb)

1 serving light yogurt or a light yogurt smoothie (11–20 g net carb),
    with walnuts added to yogurt
Zucchini Muffin (recipe on page 278) (5x5 carb)

Light cottage cheese
7 whole strawberries, sliced (11–20 g net carb)
Sprinkling of sliced almonds
"Guilded" Cinnamon Muffin (recipe on page 277) (5x5 carb)

1 light multigrain English muffin (11–20 g net carb) topped with egg
    whites or egg substitute, Canadian bacon, and whipped butter
Coffee, decaf, or tea with light half-and-half and Splenda

LUNCH SUGGESTIONS FOR STEP TWO

Sandwich of 2 slices light whole-grain bread (11–20 g net carb),
    thinly sliced turkey breast, 1 slice low-fat cheese, lettuce and
    tomato slices, and light mayonnaise
Diet drink or flavored water

Cheesy Burger (recipe on page 251) on a light whole-grain burger
    bun (11–20 g net carb), with 1 tablespoon low-carb ketchup (5x5
    carb), lettuce, tomato, and onion rings
Parmesan Chips (recipe on page 236)
Diet drink or water

1 low-carb pita (11–20 g net carb) filled with grilled chicken breast
    strips, shredded lettuce, shredded cheese, tomato wedges, and light
    dressing
Diet drink or flavored water

Chef's salad with cheese, turkey, ham, eggs, and light dressing
1 serving whole-grain crackers (11–20 g net carb)
Diet drink or flavored water

Easy Pizza (recipe on page 232); in place of the low-carb wrap from
    Step One, use a low-carb pita sliced in half to make 2 "pizza
    crusts" (11–20 g net carb)

Light cottage cheese
1 cup cubed melon (11–20 g net carb)
"Guilded" Cinnamon Muffin (recipe on page 277) (5x5 carb)
Diet drink or flavored water

1 serving light yogurt (11–20 g net carb)
Handful of almonds
Celery sticks with natural peanut butter

Tuna salad with light mayonnaise, on a bed of lettuce
Low-fat cheese cubes
Parmesan Chips (recipe on page 236)
1/2 cup Cold Pea Salad (recipe on page 248)
Diet drink or flavored water

Philly Steak and Cheese (recipe on page 256) on 1 light multigrain
    burger bun (11–20 g net carb) with sautéed peppers and onions
Cabbage Salad (recipe on page 241)
Sugar-free ice pop

1 cup tomato soup (11–20 g net carb)
Tender Spinach Salad (recipe on page 246)
Diet soda or flavored water

Chunky Chicken Salad (recipe on page 254) with vinaigrette dressing

1/2 cup Pasta Primavera Salad (recipe on page 249) (11–20 g net carb)

Diet soda or flavored water

DINNER SUGGESTIONS FOR STEP TWO

Roasted turkey with low-fat gravy

1/2 cup mashed sweet potato (11–20 g net carb)

French-cut green beans

Chocolate Ricotta Pudding (recipe on page 280)

Chicken breast

1/2 cup Pasta Primavera Salad (recipe on page 249) (11–20 g net carb)

Steamed spinach

Sugar-free gelatin with low-fat whipped cream

Grilled sirloin steak

8 Sweet Potato Fries (recipe page 272)

Tossed salad with light dressing

Chocolate Brownie Muffin (recipe on page 276) (5x5 carb)

Grilled 93% lean burger on 1 low-carb multigrain bun (11–20 g net carb) with light cheese, lettuce, tomato, light mayonnaise, and low-carb ketchup ("free" 5x5 carb)

Zucchini and Onions (recipe on page 271)

Chicken cheesesteak (with low-fat cheese) on 1 low-carb multigrain bun (11–20 g net carb), with grilled peppers and onions and low-carb ketchup ("free" 5x5 carb)

Side salad with vinaigrette dressing

Miracle "Spaghetti" (recipe on page 255) with a sprinkle of Parmesan
  cheese and lean ground beef meatballs
2 slices low-carb multigrain "garlic bread"(11–20 g net carb)
Side salad with vinaigrette

Grilled pork chops
1/2 cup wild rice (11–20 g net carb)
Asparagus spears
Sugar-free gelatin with whipped topping

Chicken cutlets with low-carb bread crumbs (5x5 carb)
8 Sweet Potato Fries (recipe on page 272) (11–20 g net carb)
Broccoli spears
Sugar-free gelatin with whipped topping

Broiled flounder
Mashed Cauliflower (recipe on page 270)
Tender Spinach Salad (recipe on page 246)
Baked Apple (recipe on page 275)

Chicken Paprikash (recipe on page 253), served over 1/2 cup al dente
  whole-grain pasta (11–20 g net carb)
Sweet-and-Sour Cukes (recipe on page 245)
Cinnamon Ricotta Pudding (recipe on page 279)

SNACK SUGGESTIONS FOR STEP TWO

Use these snacks only if an 11–20 gram net carb snack is required.

Whole-grain crackers (11–20 g net carb) with peanut butter or cheese
1 crisp apple with a dip of natural peanut butter
Baked Apple (recipe on page 275)

1 cup nonfat or 1% milk

1 serving light yogurt (11–20 g net carb)

1 protein bar (fiber over 2 g and 11–20 g net carb)

3 cups light popcorn (no trans fats) (11–20 g net carb)

1/2 cup light ice cream sweetened with Splenda (11–20 g net carb) and topped with nuts

3/4 cup cereal with 1/2 cup 1% milk (total 11–20 g net carb)

1 1/2 cups cereal with carb-controlled milk (total 11–20 g net carb)

1/2 cup sugar-free pudding cup (11–20 g net carb)

1 piece Step Two fresh fruit

1 serving whole-grain pretzels (11–20 g net carb)

1/2 cup natural applesauce

8 dried apricot halves and a handful of nuts

Sugar-free ice cream sweetened with Splenda (11–20 g net carb)

STEP TWO–FREQUENTLY ASKED QUESTIONS

How will I ever lose weight by adding carb to my diet?

With your Metabolism B, your weight is not entirely based on calories, it's based on the proper regulation of your blood sugar. Step Two strategically places a set amount of low-impact carb on top of a base of neutral foods so you can regulate your blood sugar. Without blood sugar peaks and valleys, your weight loss will continue.

My weight loss seems to have stalled on Step Two. Should I return to Step One?

During the first three days of Step Two, you might not lose weight because your liver will take on some fluid as it refills with glycogen. As long as you drink plenty of fluids during this time, you will lose the temporary water weight by day four.

Try not to obsess about pounds lost and focus instead on how you look and feel by the end of each step. The weight of people with Metabolism B will fluctuate on a day-to-day basis. Check your weight and body measurements the morning you begin Step 2 (see chapter 10) and don't measure again for at least one month. You will be pleased with your progress if you look at it over a period of time. Trust the program.

I'm confused by the five-hour rule. Is it a problem if I eat 11–20 grams of net carb in the morning and also three hours later? Won't I end up gaining weight because I've stacked carbs?

You must, without exception, eat 11–20 grams of net carb at breakfast, lunch, dinner, and bedtime. If your meals are closer than five hours and you add another 11–20 grams between them, they will stack and cause weight gain. Only insert an 11–20 gram between-meal snack if the meals are more than five hours apart.

I forgot to take an 11–20 gram snack when my meals were more than five hours apart. What now?

Every time you go longer than five hours without an 11–20 gram net carb dose, your liver releases a meal's worth of glycogen and your pancreas overresponds with insulin. As soon as you realize that you missed the five-hour mark, take the 11–20 gram carb allotment. Your liver doesn't dump the glycogen at one time, it continues until you put in the 11–20 gram allotment. If you realize that you've forgotten to take a "carb dam" between meals more than three times in a week, you need to return to Step One for a short ten-day detox to rest your metabolism. Then make a fresh start on Step Two.

I was sick for several days while on Step Two. Although I couldn't eat protein or vegetables, I made sure to eat my 11–20 net carb allotment. Is that enough?

That's perfect. If you have an unsettled stomach, use easily digested carbs such as 11–20 gram net carb crackers or yogurt, a half banana, or a half cup of natural applesauce in place of heavier carbs.

Now that I'm on a nutritionally balanced meal plan, should I continue to take my vitamins, minerals, and supplements?

Yes. Take them through all three steps of the Metabolism Miracle.

I'm constipated. What do you recommend for Step Two?

Do everything you would do during Step One—drink a minimum of 64 ounces of fluid daily, eat raw or al dente vegetables, increase your physical activity, and possibly use a plant fiber supplement. In addition, during Step Two, eat fresh fruit with skins intact and make sure your grains contain at least 2 grams of fiber.

I love chocolate cookies and two have only 16 grams of carb. Can I use them for an 11–20 gram net carb?

Not yet! Although those chocolate cookies contain the right *amount* of carb, the *type* of carb is wrong for the reprogramming phase. Cookies are sweetened with sugar and they lack the necessary 2 grams of fiber to fit the Step Two carb list. If you eat them, your blood sugar will spike and your pancreas will go into a hyper mode.

I can't seem to remember to take 11–20 gram net carb snacks between meals. Any suggestions?

Try using an alarm about four hours after the start of your last meal. Some people set an alarm on their computer, an alarm on their watch, or an actual pocket-size alarm. The alarm will remind you to decide if you will get your next meal within an hour. If not, you'll know to take a snack right then and there. Once it becomes part of your lifestyle to eat six times per day, you won't need the alarm. Routinely omitting your necessary between-meal snacks will cause weight gain and back sliding.

I have Metabolism B but my husband, who also wants to lose weight, has Metabolism A. Can he use this diet plan for weight reduction?

Although anyone can follow the Metabolism Miracle program to lose weight, people with Metabolism B get a myriad of other rewards that are physical, emotional, and psychological. The Miracle is one of many weight-reduction plans your husband can follow, but it is the only weight-reduction and health-improvement plan designed especially for you.

I've asked my physician if alcohol is a problem and she said that an occasional alcoholic beverage is allowed. Do I count the drink as 11–20 grams of net carbohydrate?

Although made from fruits and grains, the body does not process alcohol as a carbohydrate. Alcohol is processed like fat. If your physician has approved, you may drink alcohol—with the exception of regular beer, sweetened alcoholic beverages, cordials, liqueurs, and sweetened wines—on any step of the Miracle, but don't exceed two drinks, because the fat impact of alcohol will slow weight loss and fat burning. If you add a mixer, it must be water, seltzer, diet tonic, or diet soda rather than fruit juice or regular mixers.

STEP THREE—KEEPING WEIGHT OFF FOR A LIFETIME

STEP THREE BASICS

Time: Lifetime weight maintenance
Challenge: Opening your diet to more carbohydrates, including the treats that you may have been missing on Steps One and Two
Result: Keeping your health and energy levels in tip-top shape and maintaining your weight loss permanently

Congratulations! If you are beginning Step Three, you have reached the weight that makes you feel and look great. You have retuned your Metabolism B to handle carbohydrates properly and you have given your body a brighter future.

As a maintenance phase that should last a lifetime, Step Three has two key benefits: a wider range of carbohydrate grams at meals and a wider variety of carbohydrate choices. While the low-impact carb choices from Step Two will always be preferable because they are high in fiber and nutritional value, the expanded carb list of Step Three will make occasional treats a possibility. In other words, a brownie at the family picnic won't send you spinning back to detox the following day.

ONE STEP AT A TIME

Here's a recap of the three-step Metabolism Miracle.

Step One: Rested your weary metabolism by limiting net carbohydrates to 5 grams or less in a five-hour period (these were called "5x5 carbs"). You ate liberally of lean protein, heart-healthy fat, and neutral vegetables.

Step Two: Reprogrammed your rested metabolism and took you to optimal health and your desired weight. You ate 11–20 grams of low-impact net carbs at intervals of no greater than five hours. You ate liberally of lean protein, heart-healthy fat, and neutral vegetables and had the option of two "free" 5x5 carbs a day.

Now, with Step Three, you will maintain your newfound weight, health, and energy. You will identify the carbohydrate range that works best for your body, choose from an expanded variety of carb choices, and also have the option of two "free" 5x5 carbs a day. You will eat lean protein, heart-healthy fat, and neutral vegetables.

IDENTIFYING YOUR CARB RANGE

Now that you've reached your ideal weight, you will maintain that weight with a carbohydrate range that is specific to your individual body. In Step Two, you limited your net carbohydrates to 11–20 grams so that you could continue to lose weight. Step Three is less stringent, with a more generous daily carb allotment.

To identify a patient's ideal carbohydrate range, I use a classic nutrition formula that determines the number of calories a person needs to maintain his or her weight, neither gaining nor losing. Because a person with Metabolism B does not maintain weight solely by counting calories, I modified the classic formula to match the requirements of Metabolism B. When all the calculating is through, a person with Metabolism B will consume 30 to 35 percent of his or her calories from carbohydrate foods.

You can quickly find your maximum number of daily carb servings to maintain your desired weight by pinpointing your sex, height, age, desired maintenance weight, and activity level on the following table. This is a very individualized way to determine carbs rather than a "one size fits all" chart. This easy method will allow both a six foot six, eighteen-year-old high school football player and his five foot one, seventy-year-old grandma to figure out the right amount of net carb for each of them.

ACTIVITY LEVELS

Rate your activity level according to these three categories:

Sedentary = 30 minutes or less of physical activity, 4 to 5 times per week

Moderate = 1 hour of physical activity, 4 to 5 times per week

High = more than 1 hour of strenuous physical activity, 4 to 5 times per week

Carb Charts

Age	Activity	Maximum Carb Servings/Day
Teens to 20	Sedentary	8.5
	Moderate	9
	High	9.5
20s and 30s	Sedentary	8
	Moderate	8.5
	High	9
40s and 50s	Sedentary	7.5
	Moderate	8
	High	8.5
60s and 70s	Sedentary	7
	Moderate	7.5
	High	8
Over 80	Sedentary	6.5
	Moderate	7
	High	7.5

Age	Activity	Maximum Carb Servings/Day
Teens to 20	Sedentary	9.5
	Moderate	10
	High	10.5
20s and 30s	Sedentary	9
	Moderate	9.5
	High	10
40s and 50s	Sedentary	8.5
	Moderate	9
	High	9.5
60s and 70s	Sedentary	8
	Moderate	8.5
	High	9
Over 80	Sedentary	7.5
	Moderate	8
	High	8.5

FEMALE
5'8" TO 5'11"

MAINTENANCE WEIGHT OF 140–170 POUNDS

Age	Activity	Maximum Carb Servings/Day
Teens to 20	Sedentary	10
	Moderate	11
	High	12
20s and 30s	Sedentary	9.5
	Moderate	10.5
	High	11.5
40s and 50s	Sedentary	9
	Moderate	10
	High	11
60s and 70s	Sedentary	8.5
	Moderate	9.5
	High	10.5
Over 80	Sedentary	8
	Moderate	9
	High	10

FEMALE
6'0" TO 6'3"

MAINTENANCE WEIGHT OF 155–185 POUNDS

Age	Activity	Maximum Carb Servings/Day
Teens to 20	Sedentary	11
	Moderate	12
	High	13
20s and 30s	Sedentary	10.5
	Moderate	11.5
	High	12.5
40s and 50s	Sedentary	10
	Moderate	11
	High	12
60s and 70s	Sedentary	9.5
	Moderate	10.5
	High	11.5
Over 80	Sedentary	9
	Moderate	10
	High	11

CARB CHARTS
(continued)

MALE
5'0" TO 5'3"
MAINTENANCE WEIGHT OF 106–136 POUNDS

Age	Activity	Maximum Carb Servings/Day
Teens to 20	Sedentary	9
	Moderate	10
	High	11
20s and 30s	Sedentary	8.5
	Moderate	9.5
	High	10.5
40s and 50s	Sedentary	8
	Moderate	9
	High	10
60s and 70s	Sedentary	7.5
	Moderate	8.5
	High	9.5
Over 80	Sedentary	7
	Moderate	8
	High	9

MALE
5'4" TO 5'7"
MAINTENANCE WEIGHT OF 130–160 POUNDS

Age	Activity	Maximum Carb Servings/Day
Teens to 20	Sedentary	10
	Moderate	11
	High	12
20s and 30s	Sedentary	9.5
	Moderate	10.5
	High	11.5
40s and 50s	Sedentary	9
	Moderate	10
	High	11
60s and 70s	Sedentary	8.5
	Moderate	9.5
	High	10.5
Over 80	Sedentary	8
	Moderate	9
	High	10

MALE
5'8" TO 5'11"
MAINTENANCE WEIGHT OF 154–185 POUNDS

Age	Activity	Maximum Carb Servings/Day
Teens to 20	Sedentary	11
	Moderate	12
	High	13
20s and 30s	Sedentary	10.5
	Moderate	11.5
	High	12.5
40s and 50s	Sedentary	10
	Moderate	11
	High	12
60s and 70s	Sedentary	9.5
	Moderate	10.5
	High	11.5
Over 80	Sedentary	9
	Moderate	10
	High	11

MALE
6'0" TO 6'3"
MAINTENANCE WEIGHT OF 178–210 POUNDS

Age	Activity	Maximum Carb Servings/Day
Teens to 20	Sedentary	12
	Moderate	13
	High	14
20s and 30s	Sedentary	11.5
	Moderate	12.5
	High	13.5
40s and 50s	Sedentary	11
	Moderate	12
	High	13
60s and 70s	Sedentary	10.5
	Moderate	11.5
	High	12.5
Over 80	Sedentary	10
	Moderate	11
	High	12

Carb Charts

(continued)

MALE
6'3" TO 6'6"
MAINTENANCE WEIGHT OF 196–235 POUNDS

Age	Activity	Maximum Carb Servings/Day
Teens to 20	Sedentary	13
	Moderate	14
	High	15
20s and 30s	Sedentary	12.5
	Moderate	13.5
	High	14.5
40s and 50s	Sedentary	12
	Moderate	13
	High	14
60s and 70s	Sedentary	11.5
	Moderate	12.5
	High	13.5
Over 80	Sedentary	11
	Moderate	12
	High	13

MALE
OVER 6'6"
MAINTENANCE WEIGHT OF 226–250 POUNDS

Age	Activity	Maximum Carb Servings/Day
Teens to 20	Sedentary	14
	Moderate	15
	High	16
20s and 30s	Sedentary	13.5
	Moderate	14.5
	High	15.5
40s and 50s	Sedentary	13
	Moderate	14
	High	15
60s and 70s	Sedentary	12.5
	Moderate	13.5
	High	14.5
Over 80	Sedentary	12
	Moderate	13
	High	14

ONE SIZE DOES NOT FIT ALL IN THE FAMILY

Each member of this family has Metabolism B. But consider how the carbohydrate servings to maintain ideal weight vary for each person.

Dad: At forty-nine years and a height of six foot three, Joe has reached his ideal weight of 210 pounds during the first two steps of the Miracle. He runs five mornings a week for one hour before heading off to work. On the "Carb Chart," a man of Joe's age, height, and moderate activity level needs *13 carb servings a day* to maintain his 210 pounds.

Mom: Sharon, also forty-nine years old and five foot five, has type 2 diabetes but got her blood sugar under control during Step One of the Miracle and felt great at 140 pounds by the end of Step Two. Sharon takes a brisk walk every evening for 45 minutes to an hour and takes the occasional bike ride on the weekend. On the "Carb Chart," a woman of Sharon's age, height, and moderate activity level needs *9 carb servings a day* to maintain her weight.

Daughter: As a student at graduate school, twenty-three-year-old Diana has maintained her ideal weight of 130 pounds for several years. She works out at a nearby fitness center four times a week for at least an hour. At five foot four, with her moderate activity level, Diana can eat up to *9.5 carb servings per day* without gaining weight. During exam week, when she can't find the time to get to the gym and her activity level enters the "sedentary" zone, Diana limits her carbs to 9 servings per day.

Son: Eighteen-year-old Phillip plays football with his high school team. Between practice and the games, he works out six days a week for more than two hours each time. According to the "Carb Chart," at six foot one and 220 pounds, a muscular teenager with Phillip's high activity level can eat up to *14 carb servings a day* without gaining weight. As he desires to maintain a slightly higher weight (muscle mass) during football season, he then adds 1 carb serving to the 14 he is allotted for his height/weight/activity, and consume 15 carb servings/day. During the off season, Phillip still works out five days a week for at least forty-five minutes, but at this moderate activity level he decreases his carb servings to 14 per day.

WHAT IS A CARB "SERVING"?

One serving of carb is any food with a net carb count of 11 to 20 grams. To make it easy, you can think of it as 15 grams on average.

In Step One, you had to keep to the 5x5 rule and couldn't eat a full serving of carb.

In Step Two, you had to eat one carb serving (between 11 and 20 grams), making sure not to exceed five hours without an additional 11–20 gram carb snack.

In Step Three, you have great flexibility. The rule of thumb for carb servings in this phase is to spread your allotted carbs so that you have at least one carb serving at a meal or snack, but no more than four servings at any time.

Most people like to think in terms of servings, but they know that each serving averages 15 grams. So four carb servings is equivalent to 60 grams of carb, and two carb servings is equivalent to 30 grams of carb.

Now that you know the maximum number of carb servings that will maintain your ideal weight, take a look at the "Step Three Carbohydrates" list (page 126). You'll notice that all of the low-impact carb choices from Step Two show up on the list. But this time they're tallied in single-digit net carb servings rather than 11–20 gram net carb allotments. This makes Step Three easier for you to follow.

The key to Step Three is to spread your carb servings throughout the day. You'll still think in terms of five-hour intervals because that's how the liver works. And you'll have to be careful to get enough but not too many carb servings in any of those five-hour intervals. Eating too few carbs at a meal or snack allows the liver to kick in and release its glycogen stores. But eating too many carbs at a meal or snack will cause the rested pancreas to overreact. Both create havoc with Metabolism B and ultimately lead to weight gain.

To prevent such hiccups in Step Three, remember two simple rules:

1. One carb serving is the *minimum* you may take at a meal or required snack.
2. Four carb servings are the *maximum* you may take at a meal.

Although you must consume at least one carb serving at every meal or required snack, you needn't use your maximum carb servings on any given day.

Let's follow Sharon, the forty-nine-year-old mother with a maximum of nine carb servings per day. In her work as a health professional, Sharon is often rushed in the morning, has a quick lunch at her desk, takes an afternoon snack on the way to the gym, and has dinner at home. During the work week, she distributes her maximum nine carb servings in this way:

> 6:30 a.m.—Wake up
> 7:00 a.m.—Breakfast: 2 carb servings
> 12:00 p.m.—Lunch: 2 carb servings
> 4:00 p.m.—Midafternoon Snack: 1 carb serving
> 7:00 p.m.—Dinner: 2 or 3 carb servings
> 11:30 p.m.—Bedtime Snack: 1 carb serving
>   Total carbs: 8 or 9

Following the basic rules, Sharon keeps her meals and night snack to at least one and not more than four carb servings. When meals are more than five hours apart the between-meal snack has at least one carb serving.

On the weekend, Sharon's schedule is quite different. She eats a preexercise snack in the early morning, enjoys a leisurely breakfast, light lunch, and afternoon snack, often eats dinner out and has a light snack before bed.

Her carb placement for the weekend follows this schedule:

6:45 a.m.—Wake up
7:00 a.m.—Preexercise Snack: 1 carb serving
9:30 a.m.—Breakfast: 2 carb servings
1:30 p.m.—Lunch: 1 carb serving
4:30 p.m.—Midafternoon Snack: 1 carb serving
8:00 p.m.—Dinner: 3 carb servings
12:00 a.m.—Bedtime Snack: 1 carb serving
         Total carbs: 9

On a recent Monday, Sharon felt under the weather and spent the day at home, resting. She kept to the rule of at least one carb serving at every meal and snack but had no desire to eat her maximum nine carb servings. Instead, she ate one carb serving at all meals and snacks except dinner, when she ate two.

8:30 a.m.—Wake up
9:00 a.m.—Breakfast: 1 carb serving
1:00 p.m.—Lunch: 1 carb serving
4:30 p.m.—Midafternoon Snack: 1 carb serving
7:00 p.m.—Dinner: 2 carbs serving
10:00 p.m.—Bedtime Snack: 1 carb serving
         Total carbs: 6

Sharon's daughter Diana, **who uses a maximum of 9.5 carb servings/day,** normally takes two carb servings at breakfast and lunch, and three at dinner. For snacks, she eats one to 1.5 carb servings. But because of an island vacation in two weeks, Diana takes her carb allotment down to a lower range . . . bikini season!

    7:00 a.m. — Wake up
    7:30 a.m. — Breakfast: 1 carb serving
   12:00 p.m. — Lunch: 1 carb serving
    4:00 p.m. — Midafternoon Snack: 1 carb serving
    7:00 p.m. — Dinner: 2 carb servings
   11:00 p.m. — Bedtime Snack: 1 carb serving
                 Total carbs: 6

In both cases, Diana also follows the rules, making no meal or snack less than one carb serving or greater than four. She has not exceeded her 9.5 gram allotment.

STEP THREE CARBOHYDRATES

All portions = 1 carb serving (11–20 grams net carbs)

BREADS:

Low Impact:

2 slices light, thin-sliced whole-grain bread (2 g fiber or more)

1 slice whole-grain bread (2 g fiber or more)

1 light whole-grain English muffin (2 g fiber or more)

1/2 whole-grain English muffin (2 g fiber or more)

1 light or low-carb whole-grain pita (2 g fiber or more)

1/2 whole-grain pita (2 g fiber or more)

High Impact:

1 (1-ounce) slice white, whole wheat, rye, or pumpernickel bread

1 hot dog roll

1/2 burger bun

1/2 pita

3/4 ounces matzo

1 (1-ounce) chapati (use food scale)

1 (1-ounce) mini bagel or mini muffin

1 fajita shell

1 soft taco shell

2 hard taco shells

1 frozen waffle

2 (4-inch) pancakes

Breading

1 (2–inch) cube corn bread

1 ounce bakery bread (use a food scale)

3/4 cup croutons

BAGEL BONANZA

Big isn't always better. A mini bagel contains one carb serving but the standard 4-ounce bagel most Americans eat packs four carb servings!

Don't forget to count the breading on fish or chicken. The breading on most items counts as one carb serving.

CEREALS AND GRAINS

Low Impact:

1/2 cup cooked oatmeal

1/2 cup cooked barley

1/2 cup cooked brown or wild rice

1/2 cup cooked whole-grain pasta

1/2 cup cooked bulgur

High Impact:

1/2 cup cooked cream of wheat

1/2 cup cooked farina

1/2 cup cooked grits

1/3 cup cooked white rice

1/2 cup basmati rice

1/3 cup cooked white pasta

1/2 cup pasta salad

1/2 cup macaroni and cheese

1/2 cup casserole dish made with pasta

Dry cereal *plus* milk = 11–20 grams net carb (don't forget to combine carbs from both cereal and milk for the total amount)

CRACKERS AND STARCHY SNACKS

Low Impact:

1 serving crackers with 2 g fiber or more = 11–20 g net carb inclusive (no trans fats)

3 cups popcorn (light or hot air–popped without partially hydrogenated oils)

1 serving whole-grain pretzels (11–20 g net carb and 2 g or more fiber)

1 serving tortilla chips (11–20 g net carb and 2 g or more fiber)

A KITCHEN SCALE

You may want to purchase a simple food scale for bakery bread, homemade bread or rolls, and bagels. Every ounce of bread is equal to one carb serving.

High Impact:

1 serving any kind of crackers containing 11–20 g net carb

1 serving chips with 11–20 g net carb

1 serving pretzels with 11–20 g net carb

1 1/2 oblong graham crackers (3 squares)

4 slices melba toast

2 large rice cakes

8 small rice cakes

6 saltines

1/2 cup chow mein noodles

3 sandwich crackers with cheese or peanut butter filling

VEGETABLES AND LEGUMES

Low Impact:

1/2 cup corn or 1/2 ear fresh corn

1/2 cup peas

1/2 cup legumes such as kidney beans, lentils, lima beans, chickpeas, white beans, black beans, or white kidney beans

1/3 cup hummus

1/2 sweet potato or yam or 1/2 cup mashed sweet potato or yam

1/2 cup cooked carrots or 1 cup raw carrots

1/2 cup beets

High Impact:

1/2 cup mashed potatoes

1/2 baked white potato

3 ounces boiled potato

1/2 small order of french fries

1/2 cup potato salad

1/3 cup baked beans

1/2 cup mashed plantain

1 cup winter squash

SOUPS

Low Impact:

1 cup tomato soup (water-based)

1/2 cup lentil soup

1/2 cup split pea soup

High Impact:

1 cup broth based soup with noodles, potatoes, rice, or barley

1 cup cream soup (high in fat)

1/2 cup pasta e fagioli

1 cup "greens and beans"

1/2 cup minestrone soup

1 cup chili with beans

PROTEIN BARS

Low impact:

Must contain 11–20 of net carb and have 2 g fiber or more

High Impact:

Any that contain 11–20 net carb

FRUIT

All portions represent 11–20 net carb. Fruit choices should be average in size.

Low Impact:

1 apple

1 pear

1 peach

2 plums

1 nectarine

12 cherries

1/2 cup natural applesauce

1/2 grapefruit (not allowed with Lipitor)

1 cup whole strawberries (6–8 average-size berries)

3/4 cup blackberries

3/4 cup blueberries

1 cup raspberries

2 clementine oranges or 2 small tangerines

8 dried apricot halves

12 grapes

1 orange

3/4 cup pineapple cubes

1/2 banana

High Impact:

4 rings dried apples
4 whole fresh apricots
3 dates
2 figs
1 kiwi
3/4 cup mandarin oranges
1/2 small mango
1/2 cup mango

1 cup papaya cubes or 1/2 papaya
2 prunes
2 tablespoons of raisins
Dried fruit (11–20 g net carb
    serving size)
1 cup watermelon, cantaloupe,
    or honeydew

MILK AND OTHER DAIRY

All portions represent 11–20 grams net carb.

Low Impact:

1 cup (8 fluid ounces) fat-free,
    1% or 2% milk
1 cup (8 fluid ounces) skim-plus
    milk
1 serving plain yogurt (11–20 g
    net carb)
1/2 cup sugar-free/fat-free
    pudding (11–20 g net carb)

1 serving fruit-flavored yogurt
    sweetened with sucralose or
    Splenda (11–20 g net carb)
No-sugar-added ice cream
    sweetened with Splenda (11–
    20 g net carb)

High Impact:

1/2 cup ice cream (light, low-fat,
    regular)

1/2 cup frozen yogurt (light or
    regular)

OCCASIONAL TREATS

These high-impact carbs are loaded with fat and have little nutritional benefit. Still, they can be a tasty treat from time to time. They are shown in a typical serving size with its carb servings listed beside them.

1 brownie, unfrosted (4-inch square): 2 carb servings

1 brownie, frosted (4-inch square): 4 carb servings

Cake, unfrosted (4-inch square): 2 carb servings

Cake, frosted (4-inch square): 4 carb servings

2 sandwich-type cookies with filling in the middle: 1 carb serving

2 cookies, average size, homemade, such as chocolate chip: 1 carb serving

1 frosted cupcake (small): 2 carb servings

1 plain cake doughnut: 2 carb servings

1 glazed-type doughnut: 2 carb servings

1/8 double-crusted fruit pie: 3 carb servings

1/8 single-crusted fruit pie: 2 carb servings

1/8 pumpkin or custard pie: 2 carb servings

1/8 large pizza: 3 carb servings

1/8 large pizza, thick outer edge of crust removed: 2 carb servings

1 bagel: 4 carb servings

1/2 bagel: 2 carb servings

1 hollowed-out bagel (insides scooped out): 2 carb servings

1 hard roll, kaiser roll, or 6-inch sub roll: 3 carb servings

1 hollowed-out hard roll, kaiser roll, or sub roll: 2 carb servings

1 wrap: 3 carb servings

1 cup of a casserole dish such as lasagne, mac and cheese, tuna casserole: 2 carb servings

Small fries: 2 carb servings

Medium fries: 3 carb servings

Large fries: 4 carb servings

1 breaded fish sandwich on a bun: 3 carb servings

1 breaded chicken sandwich on a bun: 3 carb servings

OCCASIONAL TREATS *(continued)*

1 bun for large burgers or fast-food sandwiches: 3 carb servings

6 chicken nuggets: 1 carb serving

6 pieces sushi: 1 carb serving

1 cup Chinese food such as beef and broccoli, shrimp and veggies with sauce: 1 carb serving

Sauce: 1 carb serving

1 cup Chinese rice, white or fried: 3 carb servings

2 wontons: 1 carb serving

Breading on any food: 1 carb serving

WHEN YOU CAN'T FIND A FOOD ON THE LIST

If you search for a food on the Carb List but you can't find it, there is another way to determine its carb serving. Look on the nutrition facts label and convert the carb grams to carb servings. Using the net carb formula (see page 54), first find the net carbs and then divide that number by 15 to find the "carb servings."

For example:

Power Bar
Serving size = 1 bar
Total Carbohydrate: 46 grams
Dietary Fiber: 8 grams

46 g carb − 8 g fiber = 38 net carb
$38 \div 15 = 2.5$
One power bar has 2.5 carb servings.

Large Chocolate Chip Cookie
Serving size = 1 cookie
Total Carbohydrate: 34 grams
Dietary Fiber: 2 grams

34 g carb − 2 g fiber = 32 net carb
$32 \div 15 = 2$ **(round off when close)**
One cookie has 2 carb servings.

Soup (1 cup)
Serving size = 1 cup
Total Carbohydrate: 47 grams
Dietary Fiber: 2 grams

47 g carb − 2 g fiber = 45 net carb
$45 \div 15 = 3$
Therefore, 1 cup soup has 3 carb servings

A Day in the Life of Step Three

Let's see how several more people handle the distribution of their daily carbs.

JEFF'S STEP THREE

Jeff is a thirty-three-year-old new father. Life is a little unsettled in the house with a baby making demands, but Jeff wants to stay on the healthy road that Steps One and Two have paved for him and keep up his hour at the gym four times a week. At five foot ten, he wants to maintain 172 pounds. According to the "Carb Chart," Jeff's allotment for maintenance is 11.5 carb servings per day.

CARB SERVINGS MADE EASY

If you'd rather avoid doing the math to determine carb servings from carb grams, tuck this cheat sheet into your wallet for an easy reference. Once you know the net grams of a food you can find that number on this chart and the conversion of net carb grams to carb servings is done for you.

If your net carbs are . . ., then your carb servings are . . .

(5.5–10 gram range) = 1/2 carb serving
(11–20 gram range) = 1 carb serving
(21–25 gram range) = 1 1/2 carb serving
(26–35 gram range) = 2 carb servings
(36–40 gram range) = 2 1/2 carb servings
(41–50 gram range) = 3 carb servings
(51–55 gram range) = 3 1/2 carb servings
(56–65 gram range) = 4 carb serving
More than 65 grams of carb = TOO MUCH!

Here's how Jeff spreads out those 11.5 carb servings.

5:45 a.m. — Wake up
6:00 a.m. — Breakfast: 2 carbs
   Hollowed-out whole wheat bagel = 2 carb servings, with light
      cream cheese
   Coffee with light cream and Splenda
9:30 a.m. — Midmorning Snack: 1 carb
   1 serving light yogurt = 1 carb serving
12:30 p.m. — Lunch: 2 carbs
   2 slices whole wheat bread = 2 carb servings, with sliced turkey
      breast, Swiss cheese, lettuce and tomato, and a dab of mayo
4:40 p.m. — Midafternoon Snack: 1 carb
   Medium skim latte (using 8 ounces of milk) with Splenda = 1 carb
6:00 p.m. — Dinner: 3 carbs
   Grilled chicken
   Steamed broccoli
   1/2 cup mashed potatoes = 1 carb
   1 ear corn = 2 carbs
   1 sugar-free ice pop (5 x 5 carb, as it contains 3 grams net carb)
10:00 p.m. — Bedtime Snack: 1 carb
   1 light multigrain English muffin = 1 carb, spread with natural
      peanut butter
3:00 a.m. — Feeding for the baby . . . and Jeff!
   8 ounces nonfat milk = 1 carb

NADINE'S STEP THREE

Nadine works in an office all day and takes thirty-minute walks four times a week at lunch with a work buddy. At fifty-two years old, Nadine enjoys her sedentary lifestyle but would like to maintain her 128 pound weight on her five foot three frame. According to the "Carb Chart," Nadine's allotment is 7.5 carb servings.

Here's how Nadine chooses to spread her 7.5 carb servings.

6:45 a.m.—Wake up

6:00 a.m.—Breakfast: 2 carb

    2 slices thin-sliced whole wheat toast = 2 carb servings, with whipped butter

    Egg whites

    Herbal tea

10:30 a.m.—Midmorning Snack: 1 carb serving

    1 peach = 1 carb serving

    Handful of almonds

1:00 p.m.—Lunch: 1 carb serving

    1 low-carb wrap = 5 g net carb ("free" 5x5 carb) filled with tuna salad made with light mayonnaise plus lettuce and tomato

    1 (1-ounce) bag baked chips (17 grams net carb) = 1 carb serving

    Diet soda

4:30 p.m.—Midafternoon Snack: 1 carb serving

    1 serving light yogurt = 1 carb serving

7:00 p.m.—Dinner: 2 carb servings

    5 ounces wine (with MD's okay)

    Grilled tilapia

    Large garden salad with balsamic vinaigrette

    Broccoli spears

    Baked potato = 2 carb servings, with whipped butter or light sour cream

    Sugar-free gelatin dessert

11:00 p.m.—Bedtime Snack: 1 carb serving

    7 strawberries with light whipped cream = 1 carb serving

IF YOU BEGIN TO GAIN WEIGHT

The ease and flexibility of Step Three allows you to vary your carb intake within your maximum range and have tremendous freedom with your carb choices. Meanwhile, lean protein, heart-healthy fat, and neutral vegetables continue to be unlimited and you can still use two "free" 5x5 carbs per day. Maintaining your weight is an indication that you are eating a very reasonable amount of protein, fat, and veggies and getting adequate physical activity.

If, despite staying within your carb targets, your weight begins to creep up you need to take a moment to analyze the situation. There are only a handful of reasons that would cause your weight to increase:

- You've exceeded your maximum carb servings.
- You've eaten less than 11 grams of net carb at a meal or snack.
- You've let five hours go by without a minimum one carb serving.
- You are heavily overeating proteins and fats.
- You aren't getting thirty minutes of exercise five times a week.
- You're suffering increased stress, a recent illness, or increased pain.

The easiest way to determine why your weight might be creeping up is to keep a detailed three-day food diary that includes the timing of meals and snacks, the foods chosen, and how much of the food you've eaten. You should also note how much and how often you exercise and whether you have suffered any stress, pain, or illness of late.

When you review your three-day food diary, ask yourself:

_____ Are my portion sizes of carb foods correct?
_____ Are there gaps of over five hours without a carb serving?
_____ Did I forget to take a carb serving within an hour of wakeup?
_____ Did I skip a carb serving before bed?

_____   Am I overeating noncarb foods?
_____   Did I exercise adequately?
_____   Am I unusually stressed?
_____   Am I in pain ?
_____   Am I feeling ill?

It's easy to fix forgotten carb servings or to cut down on excessive portions of noncarb foods. As to exercise, it's a matter of making up your mind and getting back into your routine. But stress, pain, and sickness are often out of your control and can result in hormonal shifts that cause increases in blood sugar, pancreatic activity, and ultimately, weight.

You may not be able to control the source of stress, but you may be able to diminish the physical toll it takes on your body. Many people successfully use yoga, deep-breathing techniques, or positive visualization. Others pump up their physical activity to counter increased stress hormones. Work with your physician to help minimize chronic pain. One school of thought maintains that waiting too long to treat pain causes additional problems. This line of thinking supports treating pain before it gets a grip on physical and mental health.

Illness triggers the release of stress hormones that are needed for the self-healing process. Unfortunately, these hormones cause a natural rise in blood sugar that causes the pancreas to overrelease insulin, the catalyst of weight gain. Take care of yourself with rest, proper nutrition, vitamin/mineral supplementation, fluids, and physical activity to lower your risk of weight regain.

THREE STRIKES, YOU'RE OUT

Think of the above causes of weight gain as "strikes." I teach my patients the "Three-Strike Rule." If you look over your log and find that in a one-week period, you've upset the pancreas three or more times,

Daily Food Log

Time	Food Eaten with Amount

Stress Level Today:
___ Low
___ Medium
___ High

Exercise Today:
___ Minutes

Decaffinated Fluid/Water Today:
___ ounces

Vitamins/Minerals Today:
___ Yes
___ No

you've struck out and need to send your pancreas to a short stint in detox, back to Step One.

Unlike people with Metabolism A, who can just restart their diet when they stray off course, those with Metabolism B must start with a clean slate. Return to Step One for ten days in which your pancreas and liver will rest. Then progress to Step Two for ten days to reprogram your metabolism. After ten days you may either continue at Step Two or move on to Step Three.

A QUICK MENTION OF "SLIP UPS"

You're bound to have a few slip ups as you live the MM lifestyle. Twice a year—during the winter holidays and also during my summer vacation—I intentionally relax my program. After these breaks, I reset my metabolism with ten days of Step One followed by ten days of Step Two. For more on slip ups, see Chapter 8.

STEP THREE—FREQUENTLY ASKED QUESTIONS

The bottom line with Step Three is that I can eat more carbs, yes?

Yes. Designed for lifetime weight maintenance, Step Three offers an expanded range of carbohydrate. The lower end of the range remains at one carb serving (between 11 and 20 grams). The upper end of the range is unique to your situation, but should not exceed 65 grams (four carb servings).

If I decide that I don't want more than one serving of carb per meal or snack, can I live on this amount of carbohydrate over the long term?

You can. If you begin to lose weight beyond your ideal weight, increase your intake of lean protein and heart-healthy fats.

Does it benefit me to keep my carbohydrate intake near the lower end of the range?

Any carbohydrate amount within your maintenance range is perfectly fine. You needn't deprive yourself by staying to one carb serving per meal when you desire two or three. Just be sure not to exceed your maximum servings per day.

My jeans are getting snug in the waist. What's the quickest way to return to my comfortable, healthy size?

Weight gain for people with Metabolism B is not usually a function of excess calories; it is a function of excess weight-gain hormones **and lack of exercise**. Create a three-day food diary and identify what might be causing the fat gain (see "The Hit List," page 136). Once you have found the culprit, you will need to detox, with ten days on Step One; to reprogram your body, with ten days on Step Two; and then work to avoid this situation in the future.

Now that I'm on the maintenance portion of my plan for life, should I continue taking supplements and drinking green tea?

I wish I could tell you that you can get all of your needed vitamins, minerals, and antioxidants from the foods you regularly consume. In my opinion, however, because our food supply is overprocessed and tinkered with chemically and hormonally, we may be missing out on some of what we need. I think of the Miracle's supplements and green tea as insurance to make certain that my body gets what it requires.

Can I ever ease back into a "normal" lifestyle or will I be forever timing my meals, counting carbs, and reading food labels?

The Metabolism Miracle is the "normal" way of life for your body. If you eat haphazardly, your pancreas will overreact with excess insulin, you will regain weight, and you will begin to experience all the symptoms that fluctuating blood sugar once caused—fatigue, depression, anxiety, restless sleep, midline fat, blurry vision, irritability, and carb cravings. In time, you could develop type 2 diabetes and require daily medication.

Don't think of the Metabolism Miracle as a quick fix or just another weight-loss program. It is the healthiest lifestyle for a person born with your metabolism. It will keep you at your healthy weight and size on the least amount of medication.

I have two children who seem to be manifesting Metabolism B. My daughter is 10 and my son is 15. Is it wise for them to begin the program now?

Growing children require a balanced diet for growth and increased energy demands. I'm reluctant to start young children on the Metabolism Miracle program because Step One is not a balanced diet. I rarely recommend the program to boys until they have reached the age of eighteen, when much of their growth is complete, or for girls until at least two years after the start of their first menstrual period.

If, however, their pediatrician analyzes their blood with a metabolic panel, thyroid panel, lipid panel, and HbA1C and finds that their numbers point to Metabolism B, I would not hesitate to put a child on four weeks of Step One followed by Step Two, until healthy weight and labs are attained. They can follow Step Three for life with no problem whatsoever.

Your child's pediatrician should help with determining healthy weight and a registered dietitian can figure out a healthy carb allotment of 30 to 35 percent, using a pediatric calorie formula.

If their labs are normal and they are too young to begin the entire Metabolism Miracle program, you can still teach them healthy eating patterns:

- Start each day with a breakfast that includes lean protein and is not too high in carbohydrate content. Think scrambled eggs with half the yolks removed, a light multigrain English muffin, 1/2 banana, and a glass of skim milk.
- Encourage healthy lower-carb snacks between meals, such as natural peanut butter, low-fat cheese sticks, low-carb yogurt, or lean turkey roll-ups.
- Get them into the habit of a snack before bed that includes lean protein and perhaps a high-fiber starch such as peanut butter on whole wheat toast with a glass of skim milk.
- Limit high-impact carb snacks, including white flour crackers, potato chips, white flour pretzels, cookies, and candy.
- Eliminate fruit juice from your home. Let your children get their fruit requirement from a piece of fresh fruit instead.
- Avoid giving children and teenagers artificial sweeteners and caffeine. Consider using half the sugar in a recipe.

RULES TO THRIVE BY

As you follow all three steps of the Metabolism Miracle, keep the ten easy "Rules to Thrive By" in mind. Before you know it, they'll be such a part of your life that you won't even have to think about them.

RULES TO THRIVE BY

1. Drink at least 64 ounces of water and other caffeine-free fluids.
2. Avoid gaps of more than five hours without a meal or snack. Spread your food intake throughout the entire day and even into the night. Within one hour of waking up and right before bed, be sure to have a meal or snack.
3. Take the recommended vitamins, minerals, and supplements.
4. Choose nonnutritive sweeteners with care. I recommend the use of sucralose or stevia as a sugar substitute.
5. Judge the carbohydrate content of packaged foods by reading the nutrition facts on food labels and using the net carb formula (see "Easy Carb Counting," page 54).
6. Consider drinking green tea daily.
7. Increase your physical activity to include a minimum of 30 minutes, five times per week.

8. Eat allowed foods liberally but not to excess.

9. Practice relaxing. Take a few minutes each day to close your eyes, breathe deeply, shed your stress, and clear your mind.

10. Think positively! First thing in the morning and the last thing at night, remind yourself of your good health, weight loss, high energy level, continuing progress, and positive future.

Most of the rules have already been explained in earlier chapters. This chapter will give you more information on why you need to drink at least a half gallon of fluid every day, why you need to spread your food throughout the day, why you should consider drinking green tea, and which supplements you should consider.

Drink Up!

When you're on a fat-burning regimen, it is absolutely critical that you drink enough fluids. Fat burning leaves waste products that must be cleared from the bloodstream. Without enough fluid, your blood becomes overly concentrated with waste products. The brain senses this and borrows fluid from your tissues to dilute the blood. The brain then intentionally slows down fat burning until the blood is properly diluted. As you can see, it's vitally important to drink enough fluids on a fat-burning program or you will in fact slow your weight loss. I recommend drinking at least 64 ounces (a half gallon) of caffeine-free fluid each day.

TWO QUICK WAYS TO CHECK HYDRATION

Don't judge your need to drink water by your thirst. After the age of twenty, the body's ability to sense dehydration gradually begins to diminish. By age seventy, there can be little to no warning of your hydration status.

To gauge whether you're drinking enough, use the following two methods.

1. When urine is deep yellow in color, it may be overly concentrated. Check the color of your urine. If you are drinking enough fluids, it should be pale yellow in color.
2. Here's an unscientific but trusty indication of your fluid status. Put one hand, palm side down, on a table. Pinch together a little skin from the top of your resting hand and hold the pinch for a count of five. Let the skin go and see how long it takes for the pinched skin to return to normal. A hydrated hand will smooth out quickly; an underhydrated hand will return to normal slowly.

Fluids containing caffeine do not count in the 64-ounce allotment because caffeine acts as a diuretic that causes you to eliminate more fluid than you have taken in. When you drink 12 ounces of coffee, you will urinate more than 12 ounces. This leaves you less hydrated than before you drank the coffee! For this reason, I don't recommend more than two caffeinated beverages per day during Steps One and Two of the Metabolism Miracle.

GREEN TEA

Much of the hubbub in the news about green tea comes from an antioxidant in the leaves that is released when the tea is steeped. The antioxidant EGCG (epigallocatechin gallate) contained in green tea leaves has been linked to a reduced risk of breast, prostate, colon, and skin cancers; the lowering of LDL cholesterol and aiding in the breakdown of fat; the prevention of dental cavities; and blood thinning.

I recommend a minimum of two green tea bags per day (most advocates consume at least four bags per day). Steep one or two tea bags into a cup of boiling water for more than 3 minutes. Consume the tea on the same day it is brewed, to ensure its potency. Decaffeinated green tea seems to have less potency than caffeinated green tea.

WHAT BEVERAGES SHOULD YOU CONSUME?

Pure water should make up the majority of your fluid intake. To keep track, consider drinking your water from bottles or a half-gallon pitcher. Four 16-ounce water bottles contain 64 ounces. When I am at the office, I place my empty water bottles under my desk. It may look a little messy but at the end of the workday, I count the bottles and know how much additional fluid I should drink during the evening.

Other good choices include:

- Flavored water
- Flavored or plain seltzer
- Some fitness waters (check label for net carb)
- Caffeine-free and herbal tea
- Decaffeinated coffee
- Caffeine-free diet soda
- Club soda

Get your green tea the old fashioned way, by steeping it in boiling water. Bottled green tea beverages rarely contain active EGCG. Nor have green tea extracts, concentrates, or pills shown the benefits of steeped green tea.

GREEN TEA: CAFFEINE WITH BENEFITS

Consider counting green tea as one of your two caffeine-containing beverages. A cup of tea made from two green tea bags steeped in one cup of boiling water contains about the same amount of caffeine as a cup of coffee but with tremendous antioxidant benefits!

YOU MAY NEED MORE THAN 64

Not everyone gets enough mileage out of 64 fluid ounces. A large-framed man might need more; a small-framed woman may need less. In any case, drink, drink, and drink. It's a great way to care for yourself and one of the easiest things you can do to protect your health.

If constipation plagues you, take extra precautions to drink enough fluid. The majority of patients I see who complain of constipation do not drink enough throughout the day.

EAT ALL DAY LONG

A popular diet program allots dieters a certain number of points that relate to the number of calories they may use in the course of the day. According to this plan, as long as their point allotment is used up at the end of the day, the dieters are on course. Another famous diet plan cautions dieters to "avoid eating after 6:00 p.m.!" because evening calories go straight to fat. These popular theories work *against* anyone with Metabolism B. Your weight is not based on the textbook formula

Calories eaten – calories burned off during exercise = weight

With Metabolism B, you must spread your food out throughout the entire day. Eat within one hour of waking up, don't let more than five hours pass without a meal or snack, and end your night with a snack right before bed. Anytime you block the liver from releasing glycogen, you have better control of your blood glucose, insulin release, and fat deposits. You truly do have to eat to lose weight!

When more than five hours pass without eating, your body automatically lowers its metabolic rate. Alternatively, by spreading meals and snacks throughout the day, your body stays in a more awake metabolic

> Get in the habit of eating throughout the entire day on Step One to make the practice second nature for the rest of your life.

rate that burns consistently higher. Think of eating all day as though you were putting kindling on a fire. If you dump it all on the flames initially, the fire will burn brightly but burn out quickly. When you instead fuel the fire with the kindling throughout the day and night, the fire will burn steadily. Food is the kindling for Metabolism B. Eating all day gives the most steady, long-term burn.

VITAMINS, MINERALS, AND SUPPLEMENTS

The following supplements help to optimize health at any time, but they are particularly important during Step One of the Metabolism Miracle, when you are temporarily restricting certain foods. They have all been shown to work well with the Metabolism Miracle's goals—long-term fat loss, higher energy, and improved health.

Inform your physician of any supplements you intend to take and carry in your wallet at all times a list of the medications and supplements that you take.

MULTIVITAMIN WITH MINERALS SUPPLEMENT

Dosage: One daily multivitamin with minerals supplement

This supplement provides insurance that you will meet the recommended daily intake of vitamins and minerals. Women of child-bearing age should choose a multivitamin/mineral that contains iron, to help replace iron lost during menstruation. Men can choose a formula designed specifically for men. Women past menopause can use formulas designed specifically for older adults, as they no longer lose blood on a monthly basis.

CALCIUM

Dosage: 500–600 mg taken twice a day

Calcium is needed for a myriad of functions that go far beyond bone strength, from heart regulation to hormone secretion. If you fail to ingest adequate calcium through diet or supplements, your body will leech calcium from your bones and teeth, leading to decreased bone density and possibly osteoporosis.

It's a good idea to purchase calcium that has been combined with vitamin D and magnesium for improved absorption. Calcium comes in different forms including calcium carbonate, which must be taken with food, and calcium citrate, which can be taken without food. If you regularly take antacids, choose calcium citrate. Because the human body can only absorb 600 mg of calcium at one time, it is important to split your daily dose by taking a maximum of 600 mg of calcium at one meal and the other 600 mg of calcium at another.

If calcium supplements seem to constipate you, drink more water. You might also start with half the full dosage for the first week and increase your dosage the following week.

FISH OIL (CAPSULES)*

Dosage: 1,000–2,400 mg per day

Fish oil or omega-3 fatty acids help to reduce coronary vascular disease by decreasing triglycerides and blood pressure, decreasing the growth of atherosclerotic plaque and decreasing the stickiness of blood platelets, therefore helping to thin the blood.

---

*Consult with your physician before beginning omega-3 supplementation, especially if you have a low platelet level or take a blood thinner such as Wayfarin (Coumadin). Excessive intakes may cause bleeding.

WHEN SHOULD YOU TAKE YOUR SUPPLEMENTS?

Divide your supplements and take them on a full stomach at two different meals in the day, for optimum effectiveness, as follows:

Meal 1	*Meal 2*
• 1 multivitamin with minerals	• 400 IU vitamin E
• 500–600 mg calcium with magnesium and vitamin D_3	• 500–600 mg calcium with magnesium and vitamin D_3
• 1,000–1,200 mg fish oil	• 1,000–1,200 mg fish oil
	• 1 B-complex vitamin (B-50)

I recommend 1,200 mg per day for heart healthy people and 2,400 mg per day for anyone with heart disease. It's also a good idea to eat fatty fish, such as sardines, albacore tuna, mackerel, and salmon, twice a week. These fish contain high amounts of two kinds of omega-3 fatty acids: EPA (eicosapentaenoic acid) and DHA (docosahexaenoic acid).

VITAMIN E*

Dosage: 400 IU (d-alpha tocopherol)

Vitamin E has been linked to a decrease in coronary vascular disease and helps to stop damage to cell membranes from free radicals. Because vitamin E is fat soluble, you can't excrete excesses through urine, so before taking vitamin E look at the amount already contained in your multivitamin/mineral supplement. Together, they shouldn't exceed the recommended 400 IU.

---

*Check with your physician before beginning vitamin E supplementation.

The natural version of vitamin E, d-alpha tocopherol, is more active than the synthetic form. Check your vitamin E label for the lowercase *d* to make sure you choose the right form.

SLIP-UPS: BREAKS TO HELP STAY THE COURSE

The Metabolism Miracle is designed to help you reach and maintain permanent weight loss, improved health, and overall well-being. In a balanced life, there will be special times such as holiday meals, celebrations, vacations, and social gatherings when you make the decision to go off your plan for a meal or a brief time. These little breaks can be very helpful in staying the course. I always plan to slip up on my birthday dinner, my anniversary celebration, certain food-related holidays, and vacation. These are planned slips, and I know exactly how to accommodate them without jeopardizing all the positive things I've accomplished.

On the Metabolism Miracle program, those slip-ups generally fall into two categories.

1. *The party or special occasion slip-up*: When most dieters plan a celebratory meal, they usually save up calories during the day and indulge at the party. One popular weight-loss program uses a point system, allotting points to be saved up and placed anywhere in the day. You are now well aware that this system can never work with your body's physiology because your weight is not a function of calories, but of the overprocessing of blood sugar into fat cells.

In the Metabolism Miracle program, if you want to go off your plan for a celebratory meal, don't change anything during that day to compensate for the party. Leave your day exactly as it should be up until the party meal, enjoy the party, and then return to your plan that night with the appropriate snack. Metabolism B does not allow you to make up for a slip-up by changing an earlier or later meal to have less carbs.

Enjoy your slip-up meal and then return to your plan. I don't recommend allowing yourself a slip-up more than once a week.

A SAMPLE "PARTY" DAY

7:00 a.m. — Breakfast (with appropriate carb target)
10:30 a.m. — Midmorning Snack (with appropriate carb target)
1:00 p.m. — Lunch (with appropriate carb target)
4:00 p.m. — Midafternoon Snack (with appropriate carb target)
6:30 p.m. — Party (you're not counting *carbs*)
11:00 p.m. — Bedtime Snack (with appropriate carb target)

2. *The long weekend, holiday, or vacation slip-up:* For a typical dieter, it's the excess calories that cause weight gain during a vacation or holiday. For anyone with Metabolism B, it's the extra carb, lack of carb, timing of carb, and/or type of carb. Vacation shakes up your routine and that means meals may get delayed without snacks, you may sleep late, or you may eat foods whose carbs are higher than you thought.

On vacation, too many or too few carbohydrate servings cause blood glucose to rise and the pancreas to wind like a top. The best way to handle these, extended slip-ups is to reprogram your system once you're home again. As soon as possible upon returning home start a quick ten-day detox, using the guidelines for Step One, followed by ten days of reprogramming with Step Two. It's quite easy this time around:

Detox: Ten days of Step One
Reprogram: Ten days of Step Two
Back to Basics: Return to Step Two or Three, whichever you were on prior to your vacation.

I sometimes consider eating out at an unconventional restaurant as a planned slip-up. This way, I can order sensibly from the menu without fretting that the carb probably exceeds my target range. Remember to stay within your carb range right up to and after the "out of the ordinary" meal. Don't try to make up for excess carbs.

Never fret after a planned slip-up of several days. Remember that *The Metabolism Miracle* is written for you and you are meant to lead a full and healthful life. You now know how to occasionally accommodate a little food "fun" without negative repercussions. The trick is to plan for the slip-up, and plan as well for the cleanup afterward. Move forward in a positive direction, don't wallow in guilt, and get back on track so you can continue to reap all the benefits of your new and improved life.

You'll soon know the "Rules to Thrive By" so well that they'll simply become a part of your life, just as a child learns the ABCs. Follow these guidelines to help you keep yourself healthy and energized.

THE CRITICAL LINK: EXERCISE

You don't need a gym membership, expensive equipment, or a personal trainer for the exercise piece of the Metabolism Miracle. All you need is a minimum of thirty minutes a day.

Throughout years of counseling patients in weight loss, I've found that people are more willing to make dietary changes than to add exercise to their life, regardless of how important exercise is to the weight-loss equation. They get exhausted thinking about workouts even before they attempt to do them. That's because most exercise programs are based on burning calories; they stress aerobic activity with a warm-up, a workout at target heart rate, and a cool-down. This type of program is often impractical, repetitious, and unrealistic. As a result, many exercise programs start off with a bang and end up as a memory.

Keep in mind that in the case of Metabolism B, your weight is *not* entirely the result of eating more calories than you burn. Your weight is mainly a function of hormonal imbalance.

Exercise stimulates muscle cells to burn more blood glucose. This results in a lesser release of insulin. Exercise is a "nonmedicine" medicine for fat loss. In addition, physical activity tones your muscles and helps direct your body to focus on burning fat. It perks up your metabolic rate, improves mood, and helps relieve stress.

Doctor Approval

If you haven't been exercising regularly, consult with your physician prior to beginning. He or she may need to review your medications, check your blood pressure, do an orthopedic exam, or perform an EKG or exercise stress test. All of those reviews will help determine the best type, duration, and intensity of your workout.

Make It Burn

Your goal is to burn fat and maintain muscle. If you've been sitting around for the past week, doing little more than walking from your house to the car and from the parking lot to your office, then your muscle has been relatively inactive.

Imagine that your fat tissue and *inactive* muscle tissue appear dark blue. The brain cannot distinguish between the two and chooses either when it needs fuel to burn for energy.

When you get off the couch for an evening walk, that exercise causes the muscle tissue to activate. Think of it as changing from dark blue to bright red. The brain can now clearly distinguish between the two and will choose to consume the fat tissue, leaving the muscle intact.

Muscle is metabolically active tissue. Once stimulated, it burns calories for hours after the workout. The more muscle tissue a body has, the more furnaces it has and the more efficiently it handles food. Fat's main functions, on the other hand, are to insulate the body and to provide a stockpile of calories for times of famine. Fat is not metabolically active and does not burn calories at rest.

As long as you have exercised in tandem with the Metabolism Miracle diet, your brain can clearly differentiate between muscle and fat tissue—and will choose to burn the fat. If, however you decide to remain sedentary, the brain will burn both fat and muscle tissue. You will lose weight but, along with the fat you hoped to lose, you also lose valuable muscle.

Less Is More

I once had a patient with Metabolism B who followed the Miracle program with his wife. He exercised faithfully for thirty minutes, five times a week, but she opted not to exercise. When they returned in eight weeks for a follow-up, the wife had lost more weight on the scale than her husband, but she felt a little weak and tired. Oddly, he looked as if he had lost far more weight than his spouse. He had trimmed five inches off his waist, looked slimmer, and felt more energized. In addition, his lab work showed impressive decreases in cholesterol, triglycerides, glucose, and blood pressure.

As she gloated about her greater weight loss, I had to explain that without exercising, her brain had been directing her body to burn both muscle and fat tissue.

Muscle, being the heavier tissue, showed up as more weight loss. But in fact, this woman had lost valuable furnaces for burning fat. Her husband, who burned only fat tissue, which is fluffy and voluminous, looked as if he had lost significantly more.

How Much and What Kind of Exercise Do You Need?

To retain muscle tissue and burn fat tissue, you need to increase your physical activity over your own personal norm. You will need a minimum of thirty minutes of increased activity for a minimum of five days per week.

Leona, the Frustrated Exerciser

Leona, a vice president of a successful business firm, had a stubborn roll of fat around her middle and felt out of shape, fatigued, and older than her forty-six years. With her tight schedule, Leona wanted to get the most bang for her efforts and see results quickly. She hired a personal trainer to tailor a program specific to her needs.

The trainer started her on a five-day workout program with a mix of exercises including cardio, weight training, and body sculpting. Leona took the regimen seriously, determined to whip her body into shape.

Several weeks passed and the scale did not budge. The trainer explained that because muscle tissue weighs more than fat tissue, she might not immediately see weight loss as heavy muscle tissue was replacing lighter fat. Leona could live with that theory if her body looked different. But despite the intense workouts, her paunch stayed put, as if a layer of fat covered her muscle. There was no sign of toned, sculpted muscles even as the weeks turned into months.

Eventually the trainer, who did not quite believe Leona was being honest about her diet, referred her to my office for evaluation, saying, "It is impossible for Leona to eat the amount of foods that she reports, to work out to the degree she does, and have no significant results."

Leona had fasting blood glucose of 98 mg/dL ([5.4 mmol/L]; normal in the Miracle program is 65–89 mg/dL [3.6 mmol/L–4.9 mmol/L) and the doctor had flagged her LDL cholesterol and triglycerides as high. She walked into my office looking forlorn and said, "You are my last hope. I am watching everything I eat, counting every calorie and fat gram, exercising my backside off, and I can't lose inches or pounds." Sure enough, her food log showed that she was eating the calories of a woman who weighed 40 pounds less. She began checking off the symptoms for Metabolism B. She was fatigued, depressed, and irritable. She had midline fat and carb cravings and had recently suffered her first panic attack. Her mother had type 2 diabetes.

Within a few weeks of starting the Miracle program, Leona began to see the difference in her body. She kept a weekly routine at the gym but this time, as she burned fat, her muscles showed tone and form. She also lost weight for the first time in months. Even better, she regained her energy and felt brighter and calmer.

By her next physical exam, Leona's lab work had returned to normal. She has remained on the maintenance phase of the Metabolism Miracle for over four years and says, "It's not a diet, it's my way of life."

If your daily routine contains built-in activity, like that of a waiter, construction worker, nurse, or mother of twin toddlers, your body has come to expect this level of daily activity. This is your norm. You'll have to add thirty minutes of activity to your day for the muscle activation that the Miracle requires.

Some Metabolism B dieters wonder if instead of five days at thirty minutes, they can do two and a half hours of exercise in one day out of the week. It's a nice concept, but your muscle tissues need regular stimulation so that your brain will target fat cells on a daily basis. One day of activity will burn fat for that day but will not direct the brain for the next day. Move your muscles throughout the course of the week and your brain will consistently choose to burn fat tissue.

The type of physical activity that you choose is up to you. Mix it up to stimulate different muscle groups and to keep your interest. Walking, swimming, gardening, biking, yoga, light weightlifting, weight training, skiing, snow shoveling, tennis, using elliptical machines, aerobic exercise, and swimming all stimulate muscle tissue. (See "21 Easy Ways to Start Moving," page 160).

If your mobility is restricted, check with your physician about armchair exercises that might work for you, such as the use of light hand weights while watching television. If you pick up a two-pound weight and lift it during commercials, putting it down when the program returns and shifting arms for the next batch of commercials, you can easily activate muscle tissue for thirty minutes without leaving your chair during the course of a two-hour television movie.

As your body acclimates to exercise, add a few more minutes on the treadmill, a few more pounds of weight, or a few more sit-ups. Some people leave the thirty minutes intact but increase the pace. Each subtle change reinvigorates the body and keeps your exercise out of the norm for your body. Dance to another song or walk an extra block. Never stagnate—always move forward.

21 EASY WAYS TO START MOVING

1. Take a brisk ten-minute walk before work, a fifteen-minute walk at lunch, and a ten-minute walk before you go home.

2. During two hours of television programming, instead of munching through the thirty minutes of commercials, lift hand weights, do calisthenics, or climb the stairs several times.

3. Work in your garden.

4. Mow your lawn (with a walking mower).

5. Take a yoga class.

6. Clean out the garage.

7. Wash the floors, the old-fashioned way.

8. Wash your car by hand.

9. Ride your bike or walk to get the morning paper or go to the post office.

10. Work out to a thirty-minute exercise video.

11. Take an after-dinner walk with your family or brisk walk at the mall with a friend.

12. Pace the sidelines during your child's athletic games or walk the track before the game begins.

13. Bike to the park and back.

14. Swim, play tennis, or play golf (without the golf cart).

15. Take a hike.

16. Walk your dog.

17. Take the stairs instead of the elevator.

18. Play tag, jump rope, and try the hula hoop or scooter with your children for at least thirty minutes a day.

19. While on a conference call, walk throughout the conversation or lift light weights at your desk.

20. Turn on your favorite music and dance.

21. Wear a pedometer and compete with a friend to see who walks the most steps per day over a month's time.

Schedule Exercise around Your Meals

The timing of exercise makes a difference for people with Metabolism B. You will benefit the most if you schedule it around meals and snacks. These simple guidelines will maximize your fat burning by complementing your metabolic system.

If you work out first thing in the morning, eat a preexercise snack. As you already know, when you first awaken, your body is running on glycogen that the liver has released after five hours without food. If you exercise without eating, your liver will continue to release sugar throughout your routine. That will stimulate your pancreas to release much more insulin than it would release if you ate a light snack. Excess insulin will open more fat cells and cause fat gain. You could be exercising in the morning and gaining weight!

For the most efficient workout, exercise one to two hours after the start of a meal. Your blood glucose hits a peak one to two hours after you begin to eat. If you time your activity for this peak period, the muscles you activate during your exercise session will use sugar from the food and allow much less insulin release and fat storage.

Take a snack before exercise if it's been four or more hours since you've eaten. If four or more hours have gone by since you last ate, it is best to take a preexercise snack. That way you won't cross into the five-hour mark without realizing it.

Keeping Track of Your Tracks

Keep a log of your exercise in a prominent place, such as the refrigerator door. It will help you see your progress and remind you when you need to set aside thirty minutes for more activity.

Use the chart below to start your record. When you complete thirty minutes, put a check in the box. If you add extra minutes, jot them next to the "thirty-minute" check. Five check marks are needed per week minimally.

Treat the squares on this chart like the sections of a pillbox. You wouldn't skip taking your blood pressure medication, so don't skip taking your exercise. It's the critical link for anyone on the Miracle program.

FREQUENTLY ASKED QUESTIONS ABOUT EXERCISE

I don't have a thirty-minute block of time in which to exercise. Is it worth doing less?

You don't have to exercise for thirty minutes in succession. The idea is to energize your muscles for at least thirty minutes above and beyond your normal level of activity. It's fine to get your exercise in intervals: fifteen minutes or more in the morning, fifteen minutes or more in the evening. You can even consider ten-minute intervals three times a day.

I want to lose as much weight as possible. If I can skip the exercise and lose more weight, I'm going to skip the exercise.

Stop! It's true that if you were to follow the diet regimen of the Miracle without exercising, you would lose more weight on the scale. But you would lose valuable muscle along with your fat and ultimately that's not the weight loss you want.

After day three of Step One, your brain must choose to burn either fat or muscle tissue. Daily exercise steers your brain to choose fat, which is big and fluffy, and makes you look particularly heavy. When you don't exercise, your body will also choose to burn muscle, the heavy dense tissue that gives you firmness, shape, and tone.

Keep in mind that muscle cells are like little furnaces that burn fat even when you are asleep. When you exercise, you will save the muscle, and burn the fat. So please exercise.

I've heard that to get any health benefit from exercise, I must have a warm-up, at least thirty minutes of cardio, and then a cooldown. Your program is much easier. Will I really get a workout and lose weight with this program?

The answer depends on what you want to achieve. It takes at least thirty minutes of aerobic activity at your target heart rate to begin to attain cardio benefits. Weightlifting helps tone muscles and maintain bone mass and fits the Miracle requirement of thirty minutes a day, five times a week. But weightlifting doesn't get your heart rate into the cardio zone. Gardening requires muscle stimulation and also fits the Miracle requirement but probably won't get you to the cardio level. Running for thirty minutes achieves both.

Each of the activities mentioned above stimulate muscle so that the body will burn fat instead of muscle tissue. If you want a cardio workout as well, make sure that thirty minutes of your workout contain aerobic activity, such as walking, jogging, and swimming.

I cannot imagine eating a snack before I exercise in the morning. I want to burn this excess fat, not the food I'm eating before I walk!

As a person with Metabolism B, when you follow Steps Two and Three, you will use food as a way to stabilize your blood sugar and minimize insulin release. The small snack you eat before exercising will stop your liver from overreleasing sugar stores and stimulating the pancreas to overrelease insulin and open more fat cells. The snack blocks weight gain and enhances weight loss.

I understand the need to block the liver while I'm exercising. What if I exercise two or three hours after a meal, do I still need that preexercise snack?

If you have eaten less than four hours before you exercise, you won't need to take a snack. If you are going to begin exercising more than four hours after you've eaten, take an appropriate snack.

Examples:

6:00 p.m. — Dinner

8:00 p.m. — Exercise requires no snack

6:00 p.m. — Dinner

10:00 p.m. — Exercise does require a snack

I like to bike two hours after breakfast. If the ride lasts two hours, should I snack afterward so as not to go too long between meals?

Absolutely. Try never to go more than five hours between meals, regardless of whether you are active during that time. You will feel better if you eat an 11–20g snack after your ride to stop the liver from releasing at hour five.

MONTH _____

MONTHLY EXERCISE LOG

	Monday	Tuesday	Wednesday	Thursday	Friday	Saturday	Sunday	Days/Week
week ONE								
week TWO								
week THREE								
week FOUR								

Put a check in the box if you've exercised more than 30 minutes that day.

MEASURING UP: HOW TO MONITOR
PROGRESS WITHOUT A SCALE

One of the first things you'll need to do when you start Step One is to push your scale to the back of a deep closet and forget about it for eight weeks. During that time, your body will be adjusting to an entirely new way of losing weight. You will see tremendous progress and weight loss as you finish Step One, and later, Step Two. But if you stick to the traditional means of measuring weight loss on a day-to-day basis, you will suffer unnecessary frustrations.

Over their lifetime, many people with Metabolism B have gained, lost, and regained hundreds of pounds, following diets written for people with Metabolism A. The scale has always been the traditional gadget to track progress on a typical weight-loss diet that emphasizes limiting and burning calories. So dieters dutifully weigh themselves every day, coming away with a number that can lift them high or plunge them into despair.

I sometimes think of scales as "instruments of torture." Some of my patients admit to weighing themselves as often as three times a day. They remove earrings, watches, wallets, keys, and shoes before stepping on the scale. About a third close their eyes during their weigh-in and some face backward to avoid seeing the number. Whether or not they are compulsive weighers or despise seeing their weight, the number on the scale is a source of anxiety.

For those with metabolism B, stepping on a scale every day is not an accurate measure of progress. Most of their excess weight comes in the form of abdominal fat and is a result of the body's improper handling of carbohydrate caused by a hormonal imbalance. Your weight loss will have dips and pauses that will frustrate you if you rely on a day-to-day scale reading to measure your progress.

People assume when they are "on a diet" that their weight will very systematically decrease. In reality, if they plot their daily weight loss, one of three patterns will emerge. Each pattern, shown below, shows a very different outcome and can tell you a lot about your metabolism and health.

THE STAIRCASE (METABOLISM A)

This type of *plateau weight loss* is the norm and typifies weight loss for people with Metabolism A who follow traditional calorie-controlled diets. The graph resembles a set of stairs with a few days of weight loss followed by a few days without loss. While on the plateau, weight loss temporarily slows or stops for days or even a week. Plateaus often discourage dieters to abandon their program.

In actuality, a plateau is quite a healthy weight-loss pattern. It occurs when the brain, working like a sensor, detects weight loss and slows the loss until it can assess all of your bodily functions. Once it ascertains that you are healthy, it will allow further weight loss until the next check. In this way, the brain can slow starvation or allow healthy weight loss.

THE SKI SLOPE

This pattern represents *uncontrolled weight loss*. Starting weight is the top of the slope and it continues to decline, uninterrupted. Although this is the type of weight loss most people seek, they don't realize that unchecked weight loss is *not* normal. It often indicates a medical con-

cern such as hyperthyroidism, uncontrolled diabetes, cancer, or gastrointestinal conditions, and it is a red flag for health-care providers.

⟩ THE DESCENDING CURLICUE (METABOLISM B)

The weight loss of people with Metabolism B is *hormonal*. You do not
experience weight loss in neat steps but rather in a very erratic pattern
that occasionally shows you gaining weight even as you average a solid
weight loss. Because of this erratic pattern, I recommend weighing
and measuring yourself only after your eight weeks on Step One and
once a month thereafter. Note your starting weight and, at the end of
the eight weeks or month, when you get back on the scale, you will be
thrilled with your progress. In this way, you'll be spared the frustrating
ups, downs, and curlicues that occur in between.

TRUST YOUR MEASURING TAPE

In lieu of scale weighing, measure progress in inches with a fabric tape
measure (buy one at a local fabric or discount store). The inches of fat
that you lose around your belly and other areas of your body will im-
press you even more than the scale will.

Measure yourself at the start of the program and monthly thereafter.
Most people get measured by a spouse, partner, friend, older child, or
assistant at a gym. The person who does your initial body measurements should be the same person who performs the measurements
each time, as everyone has his or her own touch with a measuring tape.

Keep a month-to-month log of the following measurements.

SOLO MEASUREMENTS

If you are taking measurements for yourself, fasten the end of the tape
measure to your skin with a piece of tape to hold it in place as another set
of hands would.

Areas to measure	Month Date:	Month 2 Date:	Month 3 Date:
Neck			
Chest (fullest area)			
Women (bra line)			
Waistline			
Hips (fullest area)			
Right Thigh			
Left Thigh			
Right Calf (midway between knee and ankle)			
Left Calf			
Right Ankle			
Left Ankle			
Right Upper Arm (midway between elbow and shoulder)			
Left Upper Arm			
Right Wrist			
Left Wrist			

WHAT'S WRONG WITH WEIGHT CHARTS AND BMIs?

Americans love a good chart and we take particular pleasure, or displeasure, from finding ourselves on the spectrum and comparing ourselves to others. But "ideal body weight" charts are extremely limited and sometimes deceptive in what they tell you. I never use them in my practice because they make no distinction between fat weight and muscle weight. Some people who rank heavier on the scale or weight chart are actually less fat and much healthier than their nonexercising but physically lighter counterparts.

Take a minute and compare the statistics of two men. If you **only** look at their age, height, weight, *and* frame, you would conclude that Ray was in better shape.

	Joseph	*Ray*
Age	52	52
Height	5 9	5 9
Frame	medium	medium
Weight	178 pounds	170 pounds

The Yikes Zone

Waist	34	37
LDL	97	128
Blood pressure	120/72	142/92
Exercise*	5 times/week	none

Look a little deeper, at their respective waist measurement, blood work, and activity level, and you come to a very different conclusion: Joseph is much healthier and thinner. Weight charts that offer only a piece of the picture don't tell the whole story.

---

*more than 30 minutes/day

IF YOU INSIST . . .

If you insist on weighing yourself daily, use this suggestion. For people with Metabolism B, day-to-day weigh-ins will make no sense because the weight loss follows no pat formula. Average your weekly weights, and compare one week's average to the next week's; you'll have a better idea of how you are doing.

Look at the following example of a Metabolism B dieter's daily weight fluctuation:

Week 1 (pounds)	Week 2 (pounds)
Monday: 202	Monday: 200
Tuesday: 202.5	Tuesday: 199
Wednesday: 200.5	Wednesday: 198
Thursday: 199.5	Thursday: 197.5
Friday: 201	Friday: 198.5
Saturday: 199.5	Saturday: 197.5
Sunday: 199	Sunday: 197.5

The day-to-day loss is confusing. Now look at the difference between the person's two weeks' averages:

Week 1 (pounds)	Week 2 (pounds)
200.5	198

When this dieter compares his average weight from one week against his average weight the next, the loss is clear: 2.5 pounds.

Another chart system, the BMI (body mass index), promoted as a more accurate assessment of weight and fat than scale weight, divides your current weight by your height. But the concept has problems: It does not distinguish between gender, age, or physical activity level. Instead, it tosses everyone into the same pot, comparing men and women, young and old, active and inactive.

WHAT *IS* YOUR IDEAL WEIGHT?

Not a day passes in my weight-loss practice without someone asking, "What *is* my ideal weight?" Your ideal weight is the weight at which you:

1. Are healthy
2. Have lab work in the normal range, with as little medication as possible
3. Like the way you look and feel

When you've met your ideal weight, you are ready for Step Three, the maintenance phase of the Metabolism Miracle.

The BMI divides results into categories, with the normal range falling between 20 to 25, overweight considered falling between 25 to 30, and obesity starting at 30 and up. Using the BMI's simple comparison of weight to height, you would use the same chart to find the BMI of a young male athlete and an elderly woman. That means that you might compare a five foot nine, eighteen-year-old male wrestler to a five foot nine, seventy-five-year-old extremely sedentary grandmother.

With your Metabolism B, place your trust in a *monthly* assessment with the measuring tape and scale. If you have uncontrolled type 2 diabetes or elevated blood sugar, cholesterol, or triglycerides, you'll also measure your progress with your lab numbers. You'll be looking for these six results as you progress with the Miracle.

1. Loss of inches
2. Loss of weight
3. Increase in energy and quality of life
4. Decrease in blood sugar (if previously elevated)
5. Decrease in blood lipids (if previously elevated)
6. Decrease in blood pressure (if previously elevated)

STARTING TOO HIGH

Many people begin *this program* with excess glucose or lipids (fats) in their bloodstream. Those levels can sometimes alter the speed of the response that you see when you start the Miracle. If you are beginning the Metabolism Miracle with any of the following conditions, please read on.

Uncontrolled type 2 diabetes or elevated blood sugar: People with diabetes or prediabetes are usually familiar with the lab test called hemoglobin A1C (HbA1C). This blood analysis is taken quarterly and can estimate your average blood glucose for twenty-four hours per day, three months previous to the blood draw. If you begin the Miracle with HbA1C greater than 6.0, your body will consume excess blood glucose in the beginning stages of this program. Depending on how high your HbA1C is at the start of the program, it will take a little longer for your body to slip into the fat-burning mode. If you do not have diabetes or you have excellent control of your diabetes (HbA1C less than 6.0), there will be no excess sugar to consume and fat burning will begin immediately after day three of Step One.

High cholesterol or high triglycerides: If you start the Metabolism Miracle with elevations in LDL cholesterol or triglycerides, your body will consume this excess fat in the first few days of Step One. Once your body has finished burning those blood lipids, it can turn to your fat cells so that you can lose inches around your midline and other parts of your body.

If your lipids are in the normal range, fat burning will begin immediately after day three of Step One.

EXCEPTIONAL FARE: VEGETARIANS, DINING OUT, HEALTHY SHOPPING LIST FOR STEP ONE

Everyone has preferences when it comes to food. I see a lot of "meat and potato" folks in my practice, but I also see a good number of vegetarians and people who eat out more often than not. These patients usually express concern that they won't be able to follow the Metabolism Miracle. Nothing could be further from the truth.

VEGETARIAN FARE

The different varieties of vegetarianism all come with their own challenges. Ovo-lacto (eggs-and dairy-eating) vegetarians eat fruits, vegetables, grains, soy products, legumes, eggs, and dairy products but they don't eat animal flesh, such as meat, fish, and poultry. On the other end of the spectrum, vegans exclude all animal products, including dairy and even honey. Some people consider themselves vegetarians when they avoid eating red meat. I call that simply the preference to avoid red meat.

Most vegetarian diets tend to be high in carbohydrates because vegetarians often build their base from fruit, starchy vegetables such as corn and potatoes, legumes such as lentils and chickpeas, and grains such as whole-grain rice, breads, and crackers. All of these foods are carbohydrates.

Vegetarians who were born with Metabolism A can lose weight on a low-calorie lifestyle that excludes such foods as fatty meats, cheeses, butter, and other dairy. Their body follows the traditional weight-loss formula that says if you take in fewer calories than you burn you will lose weight.

STEPHEN: NEW TO VEGETARIANISM . . . AND GAINING WEIGHT?

Stephen, a thirty-six-year-old computer programmer, had recently decided to become a vegetarian. A self-described environmentalist, he called the office to make an appointment, telling the receptionist that he did not eat "anything with a face."

Stephen was perplexed by a recent weight gain that occurred when he eliminated high-calorie protein products from his diet. He brought a detailed one-week food diary to our initial session, outlining meals with whole-grain breads and pastas, brown rice, legumes, fruit, juices, eggs, and cheese, milk, and other dairy products.

He asked me to configure his caloric intake, as he felt that what he was eating did not add up to his weight change. To maintain a healthful weight at his height, Stephen's calorie requirement was approximately 2,100 calories per day. Yet his food diary reported that he was eating about 1,400 calories a day. He should have been losing weight on this calorie amount and yet, over the past six months, he had gained six pounds.

Stephen's new weight gain showed up right around his midline. He found himself winded when he walked up just two flights of stairs and was too tired to go out with friends on the weekend. His youngest sister was recently diagnosed with PCOS (polycystic ovarian syndrome) and his father, who had had type 2 diabetes, died of a heart attack in his early sixties. Lab work from the previous year showed that Stephen's glucose was 99 (normal is

But that's not true for vegetarians who were born with Metabolism B. They are often perplexed by the fact that although they have purposely modified their lifestyle to avoid high-fat meats (and dairy, in the case of vegans), often in an effort to lose weight and decrease cholesterol, they find the exact opposite occurring. They have unwittingly replaced many proteins and fats with carbohydrates, and of course Metabolism B wreaks havoc when carbohydrates come into the body in large quantities and in an unscheduled time pattern.

For vegetarians who eat eggs and dairy, the solution lies in balancing the diet with high-value vegetarian proteins rather than depending

---

Stephen: New to Vegetarianism . . . and Gaining Weight? *(continued)*

65–99 mg/dL [3.6 mmol/L–5.5 mmol/L]). His lipids were within normal range, except for his LDL cholesterol at 117 (normal is less than 100). I suspected that his labs had changed over the past twelve months and asked him to get new lab work for our first session. His glucose had risen to 102; triglycerides were 134; and his total cholesterol, LDL, and blood pressure had all increased. All the signs added up.

Stephen had Metabolism B, and it had begun to wreak havoc on his new *higher* carbohydrate diet. His vegetarian diet choices, while lower in calories and fat, were much higher in total carbohydrate. Grains, legumes, fruits, and many milk products are mainly carbohydrates. His Metabolism B was overprocessing these foods and depositing fat around his middle and in his blood.

When Stephen looked at the list of foods he could eat during Step One, he didn't think he could make it through the eight weeks as a vegetarian because the list emphasized meat, fish, and poultry but nixed carbohydrate, the mainstay of his vegetarian menu. He was relieved to see that his protein needs could be met with eggs or egg whites, low-fat *carb-controlled* milk, low-fat cheese, soy products, tofu, nut butters, and protein drinks. He was also relieved that he could eat liberal amounts of many vegetables.

Within the first eight weeks, Stephen had lost the weight. By the time he finished Step Two, his lab work entered the normal zone. He had been able to easily maintain his eggs-and-dairy vegetarian lifestyle throughout all three steps of the Miracle. He lives on his maintenance plan and looks and feels great.

solely upon carbohydrate. They can easily follow all the basic rules of every step of the Metabolism Miracle, enjoy their meals, and reap excellent results, losing weight and optimizing their health.

Vegans need slightly more planning to follow the Metabolism Miracle program. Because they rely completely on nonanimal and often high carbohydrate sources of protein, and because Step One is an extremely low-carb phase, I recommend their diminishing the time spent on Step One to four weeks. During Step One, protein needs can be met with soy milk, tofu, soy products, nut butters, and nuts while the pancreas and liver rest. For a vegan, it's prudent to spend the rest of the weight-loss mode, for at least eight weeks, in Step Two, which will include minimal amounts of whole grains, legumes, and fruits. Stay in Step Two until you reach your desired weight.

Step Two is more reasonable for vegans because it introduces whole grains such as whole wheat bread and brown rice, and legumes to the mix. If you are uncertain of how to adapt veganism to Steps One and Two of the Miracle, you might want to make a visit to a registered dietitian who can help you establish a plan week by week.

SAMPLE MENUS

Step One Ovo-Lacto Vegetarian Sample Menu

5:30 a.m.—Wake up

6:00 a.m.—Breakfast
    Omelet with egg whites, light shredded Cheddar, peppers, onions,
        tomatoes
    1 slice low-carb bread (5 g net carb or less) (5x5 carb)
    Whipped butter

9:00 a.m.—Midmorning Snack
    Part-skim string cheese and a handful of almonds

12:00 noon—Lunch
    Meatless burger (no carbs) with Swiss cheese, shredded lettuce,
        sliced tomato, and onion, in a low-carb tortilla (5 g net carb or
        less) (5x5 carb)
    Sugar-free ice pop

4:00 p.m.—Afternoon Snack
    Cottage cheese cup with tomato wedges
    Handful of pumpkin seed kernels

6:30 p.m.—Dinner
    Miracle Quiche (recipe on page 226)
    Large garden salad with balsamic vinaigrette
    "Guilded" Cinnamon Muffin (recipe on page 277) (5x5 carb)

11:00 p.m.—Bedtime Snack
    Cinnamon Ricotta Pudding (recipe on page 279)

Step Two Ovo-Lacto Vegetarian Sample Menu
5:30 a.m.—Wake up

6:00 a.m.—Breakfast
Egg white omelet with light shredded cheese and veggies
1 light multigrain English muffin (11–20 g net carb serving)
Whipped butter

9:00 a.m.—Midmorning Snack
Sweet Nut Treat (recipe on page 237)
11–20 grams flavored yogurt (11–20 g net carb serving)

12 noon—Lunch
Grilled cheese sandwich made with 2 slices of thin-sliced whole-
grain bread (11–20 g net carb serving), sliced cheese, whipped
butter, and tomato slices
Sugar-free gelatin cup with whipped topping

4:00 p.m.—Afternoon Snack
1 cup cantaloupe (11–20 g net carb serving)

7:00 p.m.—Dinner
3 Eggplant Rollatini (recipe on page 263) with soy meatballs (11–
20 g net carb serving) and grated Parmesan cheese
Large garden salad with balsamic vinaigrette
Chocolate Ricotta Pudding (recipe page 280)

10:00 p.m.—Bedtime Snack
Zucchini Muffin (recipe on page 278) (5x5 carb)
1 cup fat-free milk (11–20 g net carb)

Step One Vegan Sample Menu
6:00 a.m. — Wake up

7:00 a.m. — Breakfast
    8 ounces natural soy milk
    1 low-carb tortilla (5 g net carb or less) (5x5 carb) with natural
        peanut butter

10:00 a.m. — Midmorning Snack
    Soy cheese
    Almonds

12:00 noon — Lunch
    Tofu burger (containing no carb grams), topped with melted soy
        cheese, lettuce, tomato, onion slices, with 1 slice low-carb bread
        (5 g net carb or less) (5x5 carb)
    Celery sticks with natural almond butter

3:00 p.m. — Afternoon Snack
    Crumbled tofu with roasted vegetables
    Handful of sunflower kernels

5:00 p.m. — Dinner
    Spaghetti squash with 1/2 cup crushed-tomato marinara with
        Italian herbs and ground tofu browned in olive oil
    1 slice low-carb "garlic bread" with olive oil and garlic (5x5 carb)
    Large garden salad with balsamic vinaigrette

9:30 p.m. — Bedtime Snack
    1 slice low-carb bread, (5x5 carb) with natural peanut butter
    1 cup soy milk

Step Two Vegan Sample Menu
7:00 a.m.—Wake up

7:30 a.m.—Breakfast
> 1/2 cup oatmeal (11–20 g net carb serving) with 1 cup soy milk, a
> sprinkle of cinnamon, and sliced almonds
> 1 piece low-carb toast (5×5 carb) with natural peanut butter

11:00 a.m.—Midmorning Snack
> 1 apple (11–20 g net carb serving)
> Handful of walnuts

2:00 p.m.—Lunch
> Large salad containing crumbled tofu, sunflower seed kernels,
> veggie "chicken" nuggets (5 g net carb or less) (5×5 carb), and
> 1/2 cup chickpeas (11–20 g net carb serving)
> Olive oil and vinegar dressing

5:00 p.m.—Afternoon snack
> Celery sticks with almond butter
> 1 fresh peach (11–20 g net carb)

8:00 p.m.—Dinner
> Sliced Tofurkey (vegetarian tofu-based "turkey")
> 1/2 sweet potato (11–20 g net carb)
> Large portion of steamed broccoli with olive oil and garlic
> Salad with pumpkin seed kernels and vinaigrette

11:30 p.m.—Bedtime Snack
> 1/2 cup cereal (9 g net carb) with 1 cup unsweetened soy milk and
> 4 strawberries (9 g net carb)
> (total carb serving for the entire snack should be between 11–20 g)

EATING IN RESTAURANTS

Many of my patients travel for their work or simply enjoy dining out frequently. Using the same thoughtful choices that you put into home meals, the Metabolism Miracle program will work well in any restaurant. Fine dining, take-out, and even fast-food choices are easy on all three of the steps.

Step One: Be a bit of a purist during Step One. Order easy, single-entity low-carb entrées such as chicken, veal, pork, or lean steak, rather than a combination food or a choice with which you are unfamiliar. Avoid breadings and unknown sauces.

Because you don't have to count calories, portion sizes of protein choices are not an issue. You can also indulge at the salad bar, enjoying double portions of grilled veggies, lettuce, peppers, and shredded cheese, eggs, olives, sunflower kernels, and broccoli. Just stay away from higher-carb choices such as chickpeas, croutons, beets, kidney beans, fruit salad, pasta salad, and potato salad.

Steps Two and Three: It is even easier to eat out once you graduate to Steps Two and Three. You will be able to include breadings, sauces, and hidden cornstarch, counting them as single-carb servings. Just about any food can be worked into your recommended carb range when you are following the maintenance phase of the Miracle.

12 TIPS FOR EATING OUT, MM STYLE

1. **"Check Your Watch."** Consider the number of hours between your last meal or snack and when your food will arrive at your table. If it will be close to or over the five-hour mark, remember to eat an appropriate snack to "dam" the liver from releasing excess sugar before you even get the chance to order.

2. **"Have It Your Way."** Don't be timid about making reasonable requests, such as dressing on the side, an extra order of broccoli to replace the potato, or chicken breast without barbecue sauce. Keep in

mind that many people have dietary considerations and restaurants often fill special requests.

3. **"Skip the bread."** Request that no bread or chip basket be brought to the table, or move the basket out of sight so it stays off your mind.

4. **"Order simply."** Select unbreaded meat, fish, or poultry with vegetables and salad. Skip sauces, breadings, and gravies.

5. **"Make salad considerations."** Avoid carrots and croutons in premade salads, as they contain unnecessary carbs.

6. **"Replace starch with extra veggies."** Replace potato, rice, or pasta with an extra order of healthy vegetables.

7. **"Find the carb-friendly menu section."** Many restaurants accommodate dieters, with low-carb sections on their menus.

8. **"Check nutrient facts."** More and more restaurants now include nutrition facts on their menus (and some are even required by local health regulations to do so). Use the formula to compare the carb and fiber grams with your carb needs (see "Net Carb Formula," page 54).

9. **"Opt for meal salads."** A large salad with protein makes a great low-carb entrée. Choose chef's salad, antipasto, or chicken Caesar without croutons.

10. **"Request a sandwich sans bread."** Ask for the "insides" of your favorite sandwich on top of a bed of salad greens with dressing on the side. Ask the waiter to hold the bread.

11. **"Enjoy a burger with the fixings."** Enjoy the beef, cheese, lettuce, tomato, onion, and pickle without a bun.

12. **"Have breakfast for lunch."** Have a western omelet (egg whites or egg substitute preferred) with cheese, vegetables, and Canadian bacon.

CHINESE FOOD

Chinese food can be full of great vegetables and fresh ingredients, but rice and noodles make most Chinese dishes high in carbohydrate. During Step One, skip the rice, noodles, fried noodles, wontons,

breadings, and most of the sauces, which often contain hidden carbohydrate in the form of cornstarch.

Think about hidden carbs when you make an order. "Chicken and
Broccoli" without the rice seems like a perfect choice to order for Step
One, but the sauce often contains cornstarch. It's a fine choice for
Steps Two and Three, when you count the sauce as a single carb serv-
ing. Order Chinese food with no sugar or starch when possible.

Chinese Food to Avoid
Rice (white rice, fried rice, steamed rice, rice balls)
Noodles (pasta, wontons, wrappers)
Sweet sauces (duck/plum sauce, sweet-and-sour sauce, oyster sauce,
   hoisin sauce)
The crispy covering of egg rolls
Breaded or coated meats (General Tso's chicken, for example)
Deep-fried items

Chinese Food to Enjoy
Soups (egg drop soup, chicken broth with scallions, hot and sour soup)
The inside of egg rolls (don't eat the wrappers)
Steamed foods without sauces. Order egg drop or chicken broth on
   the side and use the soup as the sauce for a steamed dish.
Stir-fried dishes without sugar or starch
Mu shu without the wrappers
Egg foo yong (without gravy)
Mongolian barbecue (often present at Chinese buffets). Choose
   your own meats and veggies and request no sauce.

ITALIAN FOOD

Mention Italian food and many people envision pasta, pizza, and
crusty white bread. But real Italians don't load on the carbs as most

Americans think. I remember my parents' searching for a slice of pizza in Rome. What they found had a paper-thin crust, light tomato sauce, and very little cheese, nothing like the greasy concoction we call pizza in the USA.

Italian Food to Avoid

A tray of lasagne with a loaf of garlic bread can spell disaster for someone with Metabolism B. Instead, eat like true Italians, ordering fish or meat with pasta on the side in a small portion. Ask for pasta to be prepared al dente, which lowers its carbohydrate impact.

Italian Food to Enjoy

Antipasti. A typical antipasti platter (the term means "before the meal") contains an assortment of meats, cheeses, marinated veggies, and olives, all acceptable in any step of the Miracle. Other good appetizers include grilled, roasted, or marinated veggies, steamed clams or mussels, fresh mozzarella with tomatoes and basil, and shrimp sautéed in garlic and wine.

Soups (chicken broth with spinach, simple vegetable soup, Italian wedding soup without pasta, or Italian egg drop soup)

Salads. Most contain dark greens, olive oil, and crushed garlic. Feel free to add cheese and tomatoes but skip the croutons.

Seafood (usually great choices, as are chicken and veal entrées with sauce on the side for flavor)

Pizza. If you crave pizza during Step One, satisfy that urge by enjoying the topping—cheese, onions, peppers, spinach, broccoli—and leaving the crust behind.

MEXICAN FOOD

By nature, Mexican food is steeped in carb, with its rice, beans, corn, tortillas, tacos, burritos, enchiladas, and tamales. But there are plenty of metabolism B–friendly choices to make in any Mexican restaurant. The trick is to count your carb servings and think about what's inside all of those tacos, tortillas, and other wraps.

> One carb serving of 11–20 grams equals:
> 12 tortilla chips
> 1/2 cup beans
> 1/3 cup rice
> 2 hard taco shells
> 1 soft taco shell

Mexican Food to Avoid

Hold the rice, hold the tortilla chips. Remember to request "no rice" and shun the basket of tortilla chips. During Step Three, about 12 tortilla chips, 1/2 cup of beans, or 1/3 cup of rice = 1 carb serving.

Wraps, tortillas, and more. Most carbs in Mexican food come from tortilla shells, wraps, rice, and beans. Peek inside burritos, chimichangas, enchiladas, tacos, tortillas, and the like to see if what's inside will work for you: seasoned taco meat, shredded cheese, lettuce, tomato, salsa, and sour cream are all fine, even during Step One.

Mexican Food to Enjoy

Pass the guacamole and cucumber chips. Avocado is a heart-healthy fat and is fine during all steps of the Miracle. Use cucumber slices for dipping, or use a spoon.

Ensalada, por favor. A salad is a great appetizer choice. Skip the hard tortilla shell of the Tostada Salad . . . everything inside is great.

Grilled proteins and vegetables. Grilled seafood with a light salsa, carne asada (grilled steak with Mexican spices), and chicken dishes with grilled vegetables and salsas make very friendly fare for anyone with Metabolism B.

Fajitas. Even people in Step One can enjoy all of the fajita accompaniments (shrimp, steak, chicken, guacamole, cheese, salsa, sour cream, tomato, lettuce, and onion) but skip the soft tortilla shells. During Step Three, each fajita shell = 1 carb serving.

Machaca. This common breakfast of eggs, beef, and vegetables works for Steps One, Two, and Three.

FAST FOOD

Fast food is always a dubious choice for anyone on a diet. But you can make decent choices when you're following the Metabolism Miracle and you find yourself at a fast-food restaurant.

Fast Food to Avoid

Skip breaded chicken and fish. Although both are lean proteins, chicken and fish when coated with a breading and then deep fried take on extra carbs and fat.

Skip fries, tots, onion rings, and shakes which have astronomical amounts of carb, fat, and calories.

Fast Food to Enjoy

Grilled chicken. Along with cheese, lettuce, and tomato, grilled chicken makes a great meal.

Grilled burgers. Top a grilled burger with cheese and plenty of lettuce, tomato, onions, and pickles. Skip the bun.

Salads. Many fast-food restaurants now offer salads that feature protein, such as chicken or steak, cheese and eggs. Opt for low-fat dressing or vinaigrette.

Shed the shell. The inside of tacos works well as a meal, but toss out the shell.

EVERYTHING IN MODERATION

Remember that Steps One and Two are meant to be fat-burning phases. If you consume greasy, high-fat food, your body will waste time burning the fat from the cheeseburger before it can get around to burning the fat from you. Limit fast foods, even low-carb choices, for the quickest weight loss.

McMuffin without the muffin. Order breakfast egg sandwiches without the bread, or toss it out once you open the wrapper.

Go inside the sub. Skip the roll and turn the interior of a submarine sandwich—the ham, cheese, turkey, roast beef, lettuce, tomato, oil, and vinegar—into a great salad.

At-a-Glance Shopping List for Step One

Asterisked items (*) represent 5x5 carbs—check the label to make sure they don't exceed 5 grams of net carbs.

Beverages: sugar-free flavored water, sugar-free iced tea mix, sugar-free soda sweetened with Splenda, sugar-free hot cocoa mix, club soda, flavored seltzer, coffee, tea

Green tea bags

Supplements: multivitamin, 500–600 mg calcium with vitamin D, 1,000–1,200 mg fish oil or flaxseed oil capsules, vitamin E (check dosage in multivitamin and add separate vitamin E capsule to total 400 IU)

Protein drinks* (should have *less than* 5 grams of net carb)

Peanut or nut butter: natural peanut butter or almond butter

Cheese: reduced-fat string cheese, part-skim string cheese, part-skim ricotta cheese, part-skim mozzarella cheese, 2% reduced-fat Cheddar cheese, 2% American cheese, Lorraine Swiss cheese, low-fat cheese wedges and spreadable cheese, grated Parmesan cheese, 1–2% cottage cheese, any low-fat cheese

Nuts and Peanuts: almonds, pecans, walnuts, cashews, pistachios, peanuts

Butter or margarine: whipped butter, butter blends (combination of butter and oil), tub margarine with "liquid oil" and no hydrogenation.

Cream cheese: whipped or reduced-fat cream cheese

Meats: lean cuts of meat such as sirloin, 85–93% ground beef, ground round, ground sirloin, flank steak, London broil, T-bone, porterhouse, rump roast

Poultry: skinless chicken breast, turkey breast, turkey bacon, turkey sausage

Fish: any fish or shellfish

Pork: lean cuts such as tenderloin, center-cut loin chops, Canadian bacon, ham

Eggs: organic eggs, egg white, egg substitutes such as Egg Beaters

Soy Products: tofu, unsweetened soy milk, meat substitutes*

Vegetables: fresh or frozen artichokes, green beans, broccoli, cauliflower, spinach, lettuce, tomatoes, zucchini, summer squash, spaghetti squash, onions, peppers, mushrooms, bean sprouts, celery, cabbage, cucumber, eggplant, endive, chard, collards, kale, vegetable juice*, tomato juice*, asparagus, Brussels sprouts

Milk*: low-carb milk (5 g net carb or less)

Creamer: low-fat half-and-half or light cream

Sour cream: light or low fat

Salad dressing: olive oil and balsamic vinegar, low-fat* or light* salad dressing

Oils: olive, canola, peanut, safflower, sunflower, corn, vegetable

Cooking oil spray

Mayonnaise: light or low-fat preferred

Bread: low-carb bread*, low-carb tortilla* (5 g net carb or less)

Yogurt: low-carb yogurt* (5 g net carb or less)

Jelly: sugar-free* (5g net carb or less)

Syrup*: sugar-free* (5g net carb or less)

Broth or bouillon

Lemon or lime juice

Condiments: low-carb* or sugar-free* ketchup, mustard, dill pickles

Splenda: packets and granulated

Sweets: sugar-free ice pops*, sugar-free gelatin, light* whipped cream, sugar-free* puddings* (5 g net carb or less)

PART THREE
Exploring Health and Life Issues

THE DIABETES CONNECTION

A family history of blood sugar–related problems holds a strong link to Metabolism B. If you or a close relative has had or currently has any of the following conditions, place a "check" before the line. See "A Blood Sugar Primer" (page 194) for a description of each condition.

___ Low blood sugar (hypoglycemia)
___ Gestational diabetes (diabetes related to pregnancy)
___ Prediabetes (borderline diabetes)
___ Type 2 diabetes (adult-onset diabetes)

There is a very definite link between a personal or family history of blood sugar abnormalities and Metabolism B. If you have had or currently have hypoglycemia, prediabetes, gestational diabetes, or type 2 diabetes, the Metabolism Miracle program will work for you with success where other weight-loss programs have failed.

If you have no personal history of these blood sugar conditions but a close family member does, you may still have inherited the gene for Metabolism B. Don't wait for a diagnosis of medical problems to develop over time. Use the Metabolism Miracle program to help prevent them.

A BLOOD SUGAR PRIMER

The food you eat provides your body with fuel in the form of *blood sugar*, also known as *blood glucose*. Your body strives to keep its fuel at the right concentration, somewhere between the normal range of 65 and 140 milligrams per deciliter (mg/dL), or 3.6 and 7.8 mmol/L. If blood glucose ventures outside of the target range, the entire body, and especially the brain, is forced to run on the wrong strength fuel and health can suffer as a consequence.

LOW BLOOD SUGAR (HYPOGLYCEMIA)

There are two types of hypoglycemia. The first type, which can happen in a person with Metabolism B, occurs about one and a half to three hours after a carb-containing meal, due to the body's overrelease of insulin. Low blood sugar causes the person to feel dizzy, lightheaded, nauseated, shaky, irritable, panicky, and ravenously hungry for carbohydrate food. Within a few minutes of eating carbohydrate, the symptoms subside. People with hypoglycemia often carry food with them "in case of emergencies" and declare to their friends, "We *need* to eat, now!"

Sudden mood swings and irritability often cue their friends that they mean business. This type of hypoglycemia is considered a precursor to prediabetes and type 2 diabetes.

The other type of hypoglycemia is medication induced. It occurs when a person with diabetes who takes oral medication or insulin injections to lower blood sugar experiences blood sugar below the normal range. People on glucose-lowering medication for diabetes are strongly advised to carry glucose tablets or another source of fast-acting carbohydrate.

GESTATIONAL DIABETES (DIABETES RELATED TO PREGNANCY)

About 6 percent of pregnant women develop high blood glucose between weeks 24 and 28 of pregnancy. Diet changes, exercise, and in some cases, insulin injections are used to keep the condition under control until delivery when most glucose levels return to normal. Babies born to women with uncontrolled gestational diabetes often tip the scales at close to or over 9 pounds. These women have a greater chance of a subsequent pregnancy with gestational diabetes, and of developing type 2 diabetes in the future.

A Blood Sugar Primer *(continued)*

A TOUCH OF SUGAR (PREDIABETES)

Think of prediabetes as a red-flag alert. Also known as *borderline diabetes* or "a touch of sugar," this gray area between perfectly normal blood sugar and a diagnosis of type 2 diabetes offers a chance to prevent or at least slow down the progression with appropriate diet and exercise.

If you have prediabetes, you are lucky to have this opportunity to positively impact your medical future. The Metabolism Miracle is the only weight-loss program for you.

TYPE 2 DIABETES (ADULT-ONSET DIABETES)

Type 2 diabetes, also known as *adult onset diabetes*, comes from a combination of factors: a fatigued pancreas that can no longer produce enough insulin (the hormone that helps to ferry glucose from the blood into the cells for energy) and an increased resistance to that insulin from the very cells that need it.

After years of overproducing insulin during the prediabetes stage, the pancreas tires and begins to produce less and less of the hormone. Fat cells continually increase in size and their insulin receptors distort as a result, making them resistant to the body's own insulin. Pressure then increases on the pancreas to produce more insulin and this vicious cycle permanently impairs the pancreas's ability to produce enough insulin.

If you are overweight, inactive, and under mental or physical stress, and one of your parents has type 2 diabetes, your chances of developing the disease are high. When untreated or treated incorrectly, diabetes can cause irreversible and ongoing harm, including heart disease, blindness, nerve damage, and kidney damage. The good news is that even with a genetic predisposition to type 2 diabetes, you can improve your chances of avoiding this irreversible condition by losing weight, increasing physical activity, and reducing the stress in your life. And if you already have type 2 diabetes, you can control the condition with proper diet, physical activity, blood glucose monitoring, and medicine when required.

GUIDELINES FOR TREATING HYPOGLYCEMIA CAUSED BY DIABETES MEDICATION

If blood sugar is less than 50 mg/dL (2.8 mmol/L), choose one:
6–8 glucose tabs, or
1 cup (8 ounces) of juice, or
2 cups nonfat milk, or
12 ounces (1 can) of regular soda

If blood sugar is 50–70mg/dL (2.8 mmol/L–3.9 mmol/L), choose one:
3–4 glucose tabs, or
1/2 cup (4 ounces) juice, or
1 cup nonfat milk

After you treat the hypoglycemia, wait fifteen minutes, retest, and confirm that blood sugar is once again in the 80–120 mg/dL range (4.4–6.7 mmol/L). If it remains under 70 mg/dL (3.9 mmol/L), retreat as above and test again in fifteen minutes. Be sure to inform your physician of your hypoglycemic reaction for a possible medication decrease.

Remember that people with Metabolism B cannot lose weight and keep it off following diets written for "normal" metabolism (Metabolism A). *The Metabolism Miracle* will work for you because it was written for you!

If you or a close relative has type 2 diabetes, The Metabolism Miracle can help you to permanently lose weight, control blood sugar, and impede the progression of this condition.

METABOLISM B AND TYPE 2 DIABETES

If you have had Metabolism B without knowing it or you've mistakenly followed traditional weight-loss programs while having Metabolism B, you have unknowingly increased your chances of developing type 2 diabetes. That's hard news if you have been doing your best to lose weight and take care of your body.

The good news is that by following the *appropriate* dietary program, you can delay or even prevent the development of type 2 diabetes. And if you already have type 2 diabetes, you can use the Metabolism Miracle to diminish the impact it has on your health, by controlling your blood sugar and symptoms and minimizing your need for medications.

It's important to recognize the signs of type 2 diabetes, a chronic, irreversible disease that usually occurs in combination with elevated LDL cholesterol, triglycerides, hypertension, and weight issues. Some of the common warning signs of the disease include:

- Increased thirst
- Increased urination
- Increased hunger
- Blurry vision

Many people walk around with diabetes for years before they are medically diagnosed. Although diabetes occurs when fasting blood sugar exceeds 125 mg/dL (6.9 mmol/L), the warning signs rarely surface until blood sugar exceeds 200 mg/dL (11.1 mmol/dL). I work with an endocrinologist who automatically tacks five years onto the date of a person's diabetes diagnosis. He believes that it takes about five years from when blood sugar initially exceeds 125 mg/dL to when that person feels ill and seeks medical attention.

A diagnosis of type 2 diabetes is usually made when two fasting blood glucose readings are shown to be *more than* 126 mg/dL (7 mmol/L).

	Normal	*Prediabetes*	*Type 2 Diabetes*
Fasting blood sugar (in mg/dL)	65–99	100–125	*greater than* 126*
2 hours after eating (in mg/dL)	less than 140	greater than 140 but less than 200	greater than 200

Type 2 diabetes carries the potential for a number of life-threatening health consequences down the road, including blindness, kidney failure, heart attack, stroke, amputation, and nerve disorders. To understand how years of high blood glucose cause so much damage, you must look inside the blood vessels.

Regardless of what they eat or drink, the blood sugar of a person without glucose problems will never exceed 140 mg/dL (7.8 mmol/L). By contrast, people with prediabetes or diabetes frequently have blood glucose above 140. This supersaturated blood sugar paints the lining of every blood vessel with a syrupy coating.

The sticky, sugar-coated walls of blood vessels act like glue for excess LDL and triglycerides. Remember that people with untreated Metabolism B typically have elevated blood lipids. It's no wonder that a person with type 2 diabetes has a 50 percent greater chance of suffering a heart attack or stroke than does a nondiabetic person. The thicker the deposits of fat become, the narrower the diameter of the blood vessel. Eventually, the individual accumulates a significant blockage that can ultimately lead to a heart attack or stroke.

In addition, blood vessels should be flexible and bend like a well-cooked strand of spaghetti. The blood vessels of a person with uncontrolled diabetes will harden and may break or have jagged edges that

---

*Type 2 diabetes is most often diagnosed by fasting blood glucose.

catch circulating fats like a dam blocks a stream and cause inflammation that has been linked to heart disease.

It is this damage to the blood vessels and nerves that leads to each of the following health-threatening complications of diabetes.

Retinopathy: When tiny blood vessels in the retina of the eye harden and eventually break and hemorrhage that can lead to blindness.

Neuropathy: Nerve endings that have been exposed to high levels of sugar for a period of time can harden, decreasing the nerve's ability to transfer impulses. Such damage can lead to hypersensation, lack of sensation, digestive problems, irregular heartbeat, sexual dysfunction, and more.

Nephropathy: Year after year, elevated blood sugar hardens the small blood vessels of the kidney, causing them to snap. Broken blood vessels impede the kidney's ability to filter toxins from the blood. As filtering ability decreases, toxins and waste products build up in the blood and may lead to the need for renal dialysis.

Circulatory Problems: Because your feet contain the vessels furthest from the heart, vessel damage from plaque and hardening impede circulation and deaden nerves. Antibiotics may not be able to reach an infection in the feet and legs. Serious circulatory problems can lead to amputations.

It's All about Control

Complications from diabetes occur *only* when the disease goes uncontrolled. The Metabolism Miracle gives you the knowledge and skills to control the two main components of type 2 diabetes—insulin resistance and a burned-out pancreas.

People with Metabolism B are born with a genetic propensity to overrelease insulin in response to a rise in blood sugar. Remember that

First Things First

Before beginning any diet or exercise program, contact your physician. This is particularly important if you have diabetes and are taking oral medication or insulin to control blood sugar. *The Metabolism Miracle* will help you to lose weight and decrease blood sugar, blood pressure, and blood lipids, and those changes may warrant a change in your medication or dosage.

Keep your doctor abreast of weight losses of 10 pounds or more and always report symptoms that might indicate overmedication.

insulin is the hormone responsible for ferrying blood glucose into the muscle and fat cells of the body. When an event or hormonal change in the life of someone with Metabolism B triggers the pancreas to manifest this hyperinsulin release, it eventually leads to weight gain. The more weight that people with Metabolism B gain, the higher their risk of developing insulin resistance.

As you gain weight, your fat cells get larger in size. When you lose weight, they decrease in size. Both fat and muscle cells have receptors for insulin to attach and open the cell for glucose. Insulin acts like a key, fitting the receptor keyholes. The insulin receptors of people with Metabolism A will remain constant in shape no matter how large their fat cells become. But when people with Metabolism B gain weight, the fat cells stretch and their insulin receptors warp to the point that the key no longer fits the keyhole. When this happens, such people are now resistant to their own insulin.

The cell sends a message to the brain that it is hungry and needs insulin to open its door and usher in the glucose. The brain keeps calling on the pancreas to release insulin. The pancreas obliges, but because the insulin keys can't fit properly into the keyhole receptors, the glucose rarely gets into the cell. The brain calls on the pancreas over and over again. Eventually the pancreas fatigues to the point of exhaustion, cells are underfed, sugar backs up in the bloodstream, and you have the beginning of type 2 diabetes.

STOP THE TRAIN

Think of type 2 diabetes as a runaway train. It is best to stop the train in its tracks as early as possible. When detected early, diabetes can be successfully treated with diet and exercise. Unfortunately, the traditional diet for diabetes will speed up the pancreas burn out and the stretching of the insulin receptors. The traditional American Diabetes Association diet recommends a meal plan that contains about 50 to 55 percent carbohydrate. As you know, 100 percent of carbohydrate converts to blood sugar and causes the pancreas to release insulin. The main nutrient in the traditional diet for diabetes is the one nutrient that the person with diabetes cannot handle effectively.

When traditional diet fails to control blood sugar in type 2 diabetes, the next step is to take oral medications. Keep in mind that the traditional diet overworks the pancreas with its excessive amount of carbohydrate. The oral diabetes medications that can lower blood glucose are medications that force the pancreas to release even more insulin. The very medication prescribed to lower blood sugar is medication that will speed up the burn out of the pancreas. Once the pancreas is burned out, no amount of oral medication can squeeze more insulin from the pancreas. At this point, the only option is injecting insulin for the rest of the person's life.

There is a way to stop the train. If you have Metabolism B and follow the Metabolism Miracle program as a way of life, you will absolutely lose weight. Your pancreas will rest before it is irretrievably burned out. You will retrain your pancreas to react normally to blood glucose changes. As you lose weight, your insulin receptors will regain their original shape. You can prevent or greatly forestall the onset of type 2 diabetes. If you already have type 2 diabetes, and you follow the Metabolism Miracle way of life, you can actually prevent complications or forestall the need for insulin injections, effectively stopping the runaway metabolic train in its tracks.

WILL EVERY PERSON WITH METABOLISM B DEVELOP TYPE 2 DIABETES?

For a long time, the medical community thought that type 2 diabetes, hypertension, and high cholesterol came as the direct result of overeating and lack of physical activity. We now know that the genetic predisposition for excess insulin release and insulin resistance starts this process for people with Metabolism B.

Everyone with Metabolism B has the *potential* to develop type 2 diabetes, but not everyone will. You cannot develop type 2 diabetes without the genetic predisposition for the disease—the same predisposition as Metabolism B. Think of diabetes as the last stop of the Metabolism B train. It appears that a combination of being born with the gene and environmental stressors moves the train through the stops of midline weight, to elevated blood pressure, to elevated lipids, to elevated blood sugar and to type 2 diabetes. When a person who is born with Metabolism B is exposed to certain environmental triggers, his or her chances of developing type 2 diabetes will increase.

The greater the number of environmental factors that the person with Metabolism B is exposed to, the greater are his or her chances of developing diabetes.

When a person is diagnosed with type 2 diabetes, his or her midline weight is often at its highest point, coupled with physical activity at an all-time low. Stress may have recently increased or been occurring for an extended period of time. Add an illness as fleeting as a flu to the mix, and the chance of the symptoms progressing goes up even further.

THE DIABETES SETUP

This chart lists the combination of factors that conspire to trigger type 2 diabetes. If you have the gene for Metabolism B, any of the following environmental factors may usher you toward developing type 2 diabetes.

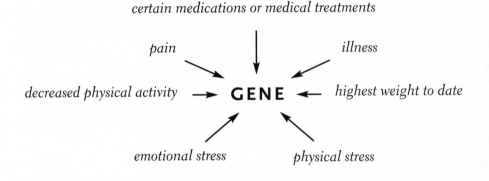

certain medications or medical treatments

pain   illness

decreased physical activity → **GENE** ← highest weight to date

emotional stress   physical stress

Given the conditions that may trigger diabetes, it makes wise sense for anyone with Metabolism B and thus the chance of developing type 2 diabetes, to reduce weight with the appropriate diet, increase physical activity, learn to manage stress, and stay as healthy as possible.

The Metabolism Miracle helps you to beat the odds.

TRANSFORMATIONS: STORIES FROM THE FIELD

One of the truths about Metabolism B is that it affects so many different types of people, in so many different walks of life. I've seen thousands of patients over the past twenty-five years and since the development of this program I've watched a lot of transformations take place as the Metabolism Miracle begins to work its magic. The following stories represent just a few of the many different people whom this program has helped usher from despair to empowerment.

MARGE, THE RETIRED NURSE

After years of procrastinating, sixty-nine-year-old Marge, a retired nurse, visited her orthopedic specialist to set up a date for knee replacement surgery. Marge had always been active, spending most of her working life on her feet. As a nurse at the community hospital she stood for hours and felt the effects on her spine and joints. Still, she was surprised to learn that over the years her "good" knee had also deteriorated and she would require double knee replacements. To make matters worse, the doctor informed Marge that her blood sugar was borderline high and her blood pressure was slightly elevated.

Over the years, Marge had put on a few pounds and realized that the extra weight didn't help her joint pain. She attributed the weight gain to aging and the slower pace of her retired life. She hadn't worried about her weight until the surgeon told her to lose twenty pounds before he would operate.

Marge hobbled into my office, using a cane. She appeared older than her years and walked bent over with a limp, obviously in pain. She knew weight loss would help her properly rehabilitate after surgery but didn't know where to begin. She couldn't possibly exercise at this time and didn't see herself cooking elaborate meals or buying special foods.

Based on her diagnosis of prediabetes and hypertension, we decided the Metabolism Miracle matched her metabolism and would help her to lose weight quickly and permanently. It could also prevent her progression to type 2 diabetes, and the weight loss would help to lower her blood pressure.

I explained that meal preparation need not be cumbersome and that many foods required very little preparation, such as an egg white omelet with low-carb toast, a wrap with tuna, a protein shake and a handful of almonds, or cottage cheese and veggies or low-carb yogurt with a Miracle-recipe muffin. Marge would exercise using light hand weights and do muscle-toning activities in an armchair until the physical therapy after surgery. She was pleased to learn that it wasn't about how many calories burned, it was about energizing muscle tissue.

After Step One and eight weeks on Step Two with a weight loss of twenty-two pounds, Marge had her double knee replacement and began physical therapy until she was navigating independently. The recovery had interrupted her normal diet and so Marge returned to ten days of Step One, followed by Step Two until she reached her desired weight. She is now cane-free, pain-free, and remains diabetes-free. She uses Step Three, the maintenance phase of the Miracle, with brief intervals of Steps One and Two, to give her system an occasional cleansing.

DAVE, THE HIGH SCHOOL ATHLETE

When Dave first came to my practice, he was a junior in high school. An honor student and member of both the baseball and football teams, Dave was generally upbeat, motivated, and, although quiet, he enjoyed hanging out with his many friends.

At five foot ten and 185 pounds, Dave lifted weights between sports seasons and always considered himself to be "tight and muscular." He reported eating everything and anything, including favorite foods such as bagels, pizza, chicken fingers, subs, Chinese food, burgers, and fries, always washed down with a cola or iced tea.

After football season junior year, Dave noticed he felt much less energetic. His parents figured that his long days, school, homework, and friends caused the problem. Dave knew it was more than that. He had trouble waking up and felt wiped out after breakfast, after lunch, when he got home from school, and after dinner. It seemed as if he sank every time he ate a meal. He also, for the first time, had difficulty concentrating in class. Along with the fatigue, his mind wandered. He couldn't pay attention to lessons and even after studying he had difficulty recalling the information for exams. He began to depend upon energy drinks in the evening to help him stay focused. When his third-quarter grades arrived, it was obvious something was wrong. His grades had dropped from the honor roll to include several Cs.

In the weight room, Dave also felt the drain. He had less energy to lift weights before baseball season and noticed that his belly had begun to protrude. One of his friends remarked that Dave was getting a gut. He felt more interested in watching sports from the couch than he did about going to the batting cages to get ready for the season.

Concerned about his slumping grades and his unusual choice of choosing video games and television over being with his friends or playing sports, his mother scheduled an appointment with Dave's doctor. After some prodding, Dave told his doctor that he was drained, down in the dumps, had no desire to do the things he used to enjoy, and was having difficulty in school. On the surface this sounded like mild depression, but after ruling out mononucleosis and Lyme disease, lab tests revealed surprises for the physician. This young, athletic male had a fasting glucose of 115 mg/dL (normal is 65–99 mg/dL or 3.6–5.5 mmol/L), total cholesterol of 212 (normal is less than 200) and LDL cholesterol of 118 (normal is less than 100).

Dave came to my office with a diagnosis of prediabetes and hyperlipidemia. He also had a teenager's skepticism. But he did recognize Metabolism B in himself as we discussed his symptoms of fatigue, anxiety, poor short-term memory, belly fat, and irritability. Mostly he wanted his old life back. He promised to "give it a shot" but, as he left my office, I wondered if he was being sincere.

Step One was a challenge to a young man who ate out with friends on a regular basis. He explained to buddies that he was on a boot camp–style program. They thought it was cool that Dave could use his diet and exercise to resculpt and rebuild his body. He never mentioned to them that the real reason for his lifestyle change was elevated cholesterol, high blood sugar, and a growing midline paunch. Dave chose from any menu that came his way; even fast-food menus had possibilities. At the local fast-food joint, he'd order two large grilled burgers "his way" with cheese, tomato slices, onions, pickles, and no bun. He even asked for extra lettuce in place of the bun and could pick up his huge creation with no problem! A sugar-free soda capped the meal. If he was still hungry, he'd also order a chicken Caesar side salad in place of his fries. He loved the freedom of liberal portions of lean protein, healthy fat, vegetables, and protein shakes.

Within a few weeks Dave felt and looked better. His friends, and most important, his girlfriends, told him he looked great. He could already see the difference in his ability to concentrate and he felt like his old self.

Over the summer, Dave completed Step Two, reentering a world in which he enjoyed hanging out with friends and playing Frisbee on the beach. He began his senior year on Step Three, maintenance, and he says he has permanently adopted the Miracle not as a diet but as a way of life. He intends to live his life healthy and happy.

KAREN AND THE WEIGHT OF FAMILY BAGGAGE

Karen, who was referred to my practice by her psychiatrist, was overweight as a child and remembers "being on a diet" since she was about seven years old. She has clear memories of her mother calling her chubby and critiquing her food choices in front of friends and family. To this day, she feels the tension with her mother and can't shed the feeling of that embarrassed, chubby child when she visits her parents' home.

When Karen went away to college, she was able to take control of her weight. She juggled work, school, and a busy lifestyle. Without a car, she walked everywhere on campus. She was known for her upbeat, sunny, positive personality and felt on top of the world and in control of her weight and life.

After graduation she became a third grade teacher and married her college sweetheart. On the outside, her world appeared perfect: a bright, healthy, happy, married woman embarking on life and career.

But something changed in December of her first year as a teacher. Karen felt decidedly different. She woke up exhausted, even after enough sleep. She stopped for a bagel on the way to work but needed coffee to give her some zip. She began to feel anxious on the way to work and sometimes felt her heart race and a cold sweat form on her face before entering the classroom.

Right before recess, she would begin to feel shaky and found herself watching the clock hoping she could make it until the bell rang. As soon as the children filed out of the classroom, she hurriedly ate a candy bar from her purse. The behavior embarrassed her but she couldn't seem to control it. The same feeling happened when she came home from school in the afternoon. She found herself in the kitchen, opening cabinet after cabinet, eating a little of this and a little of that. Next came the refrigerator, and Karen couldn't stop herself from consuming anything—peanut butter, cheese, cake, or leftovers. She knew that this was not normal but she couldn't stop.

After her afternoon binges, disgusted with what she had done, Karen would need a nap, and she noticed that after dinner she had to lie down again because of how wiped out she felt. Her husband washed the dishes and cleaned up the kitchen while Karen dozed in front of the television. When he went to bed for the night, she would wake up and snack again.

One morning before her shower, Karen was shocked by her reflection in the bathroom mirror. How had she not noticed her belly, love handles, and back fat? Why hadn't anyone told her? But that was exactly what she despised about her childhood: being reminded of her weight gain. She realized at that moment that she had a problem and needed help.

Karen made an appointment with a psychiatrist and a medical doctor who ordered lab work before he began working with her. He found tell-tale signs: her glucose was 104 (normal is 65–99 mg/dL or 3.6–5.5 mmol/L), and her triglycerides, LDL cholesterol, and HbA1C were all elevated. Karen was dealing with a physical problem along with her psychological problems. He referred her to my office to learn about her dietary needs based on her metabolism. Until her excess insulin and insulin resistance were treated and her metabolism stabilized, no amount of psychotherapy could help.

Karen was thrilled to understand the physical reasons for her eating behaviors and eagerly made the diet and exercise changes on the Miracle. Now her lab numbers are under control and, working in tandem with her psychiatrist, Karen has reached her desired weight and come to terms with how her childhood has affected her body image and eating patterns. She and her husband hope to have a child soon, so we will next meet to tailor her program for pregnancy and lactation.

JIM, TYPE 2 DIABETES AND A HOVERING WIFE

When Jim's wife, Barbara, called my office to make an appointment for her husband, she sounded anxious and reported that she was "at the end of her rope" with Jim, who had recently retired and now spent much of his time at home.

Jim, a salesman who traveled from city to city, was self-motivated and independent and had been very effective in his job. Now that they spent almost every waking hour together, Barbara worried about how her husband took care of himself and was concerned about their future. For the first time since Jim's diagnosis with type 2 diabetes ten years before, Barbara could witness his entire day, from wakeup to bedtime.

Barbara walked into the office first, with Jim walking behind. She filled in the initial assessment form while Jim read *Newsweek*. She pulled his medication list from her wallet and asked the receptionist to make a copy for his chart.

The couple's dynamic continued during the beginning of Jim's initial session. Barbara had a copy of her husband's daily blood sugar log. Although I tried to direct the questions to him, his wife finished his sentences and filled in the gaps of his diet history. About 30 minutes into our session, Barbara left for the restroom. While she was gone, I asked Jim if he would mind if we spoke about his diabetes care one-on-one. He didn't seem to care either way. Barbara waited in the reception room.

Without interruption or distraction, Jim and I worked very well together. It often helps to explain diabetes in a very concrete way, using the analogy of the body as a car and the problems that would occur if the car was forced to run on diesel instead of unleaded fuel. Like keeping up a car's maintenance, Jim needed to check his blood sugar at least twice a day, fill the tank with the appropriate fuel (carb allotment), run the car daily (exercise), and keep records of maintenance (log book/food log). My job was to teach him to take the best care of his health so that he would "run smoothly" for many years to come.

Jim's maintenance plan included checking his blood sugar twice a day, logging his results, and thinking of possible explanations for the readings (food, lack of exercise, forgotten medication, or stress). He would also walk for thirty minutes daily and begin Step One of the Miracle. Since Barbara was in charge of the household's shopping, menus, and meal preparation, we invited her back into the session.

Jim explained that he was going to take care of the monitoring, exercise, logging, and medication, and that he would like Barbara's help as they got acclimated to Step One of the program. Barbara seemed both relieved and put out that she would not be totally involved in the management of Jim's diabetes.

Jim e-mailed me his blood sugar readings on a weekly basis, with notations for exercise and the reasons he felt readings were out of range. A weekly food log showed that he was on target with his diet program. Occasionally, Barbara would e-mail a few questions. She also made note that Jim was in control and feeling and looking much better.

When the couple returned in eight weeks for follow-up, Jim held the door open for Barbara, filled in his follow-up form, and handed me his records. While he had learned what he needed to do to maintain his health and well-being, Barbara had learned to support Jim in his self-management and attended his sessions as a "second set of ears."

As time passed, Jim's doctor adjusted his medication for diabetes, based on his much improved blood sugar. He now maintains excellent blood sugar while living on Step Three of the Metabolism Miracle. He does daily physical activity, takes much less medication, and enjoys a less stressful home life.

ANDREA, 25 YEARS OLD AND CONSIDERING GASTRIC BYPASS SURGERY

Three years ago, a young woman appeared at my office to fulfill her surgeon's requirement that she meet with a registered dietitian before she could be scheduled for gastric bypass surgery.

Andrea was visibly upset. She made very little eye contact and seemed ashamed to find herself in this position. As we talked, she told me of her years as a track star at high school and the track scholarship she received that enabled her to attend a top university. During her junior year, she suffered an orthopedic injury that required several surgeries and abruptly ended her days of training and competing. Over the past four years, she had gained ninety-five pounds.

At twenty-five years of age, Andrea was five foot six. In her running days, she competed at a weight of 150 pounds, but with her muscular body she'd appeared much thinner. She asked if she could face backward when I got her initial weight, as she couldn't bear to see the scale. Because she had lost much of her muscle tissue and tone, she appeared even heavier than her current 245 pounds.

Andrea had assumed that her tremendous weight gain had happened because of her lack of exercise, since her diet hadn't changed much since college. Yet she still used a treadmill for thirty minutes three to four times a week. She had put genuine effort and time into four very

THE MYTH OF GASTRIC BYPASS

Gastric bypass surgery is a weight-loss surgical procedure that physically rewires the digestive system. The stomach is cut and stapled so a remaining 2-ounce pouch limits the amount of food a person can eat at one time. The small intestine is also cut and reattached to the newly formed stomach pouch. The duodenum of the small intestine is literally bypassed.

This bypass of the first portion of the small intestine prevents the patient from absorbing all the nutrients out of the small amount of food that can still fit in the tiny pouch. As time passes, the stomach pouch stretches in size. After about a year and a half, the pouch has an 8-ounce capacity.

At about the one-and-a-half-year to two-year mark after gastric bypass surgery, those with Metabolism B usually note that their weight loss abruptly stops. Right after that, they start to slowly but surely regain weight. Although the surgery bypasses the duodenum of the small intestine, it does not bypass the genes for Metabolism B. Ironically, these patients end up needing to follow the Metabolism Miracle after having permanently rewired their GI tract.

popular diet approaches before giving up and deciding to go for the bypass. She was tired of dieting and gaining weight. She was tired of failing. She was tired of feeling tired. Andrea was resigned to do the surgery, deal with the possible side effects, and move on with her life.

We assessed Andrea's symptoms. Her grandmother had type 2 diabetes and her father, who took medication for high cholesterol and high blood pressure, was recently warned to "watch his sugar." Andrea carried a good portion of her weight around her middle. She complained about being depressed and about the way she looked and felt. She recently suffered a panic attack and cried easily. She described herself as a carb addict, craved crunchy foods and chocolate, and couldn't seem to stop eating because she never felt full. She recently began to drink coffee for energy.

Andrea's fasting lab data showed a blood glucose level of 101 (normal is 65–99 md/dL or 3.6–5.5 mmol/L), total cholesterol of 197 (normal is less than 200), LDL cholesterol of 130 (normal is less than 100), and HDL "good" cholesterol of 35 (normal is greater than 45). She had a history of irregular, heavy, clotty periods.

It was clear to me, given her rapid weight gain, placement of fat on her body, family history of diabetes and metabolic syndrome, symptoms, and lab work that she had Metabolism B and could benefit hugely from the Miracle. Andrea, however, had come to my office to check off the "I met with the dietitian box" on her presurgery questionnaire.

I told Andrea that gastric bypass is a permanent rearrangement of the GI tract but it does not bypass the genes for Metabolism B. She might lose a hundred pounds in a year, but as soon as the stomach stretches to a certain capacity (about eight ounces), carb intake can again trip up the pancreas's hyperactivity and cause weight gain. I see many patients at less than two years after this major surgery, to teach the Metabolism Miracle for weight reduction. They have had a permanent gastric bypass and end up on the very same diet they could have followed before such a drastic measure was taken.

I asked Andrea to consider giving my program a four-month chance. If, at the end of four months, she still wanted to go on with the surgery, I would understand. Andrea decided to give the Metabolism Miracle a chance with the understanding that if it didn't work for her, I would clear her dietarily for the surgery. I planned to see her at the eight-week, twelve-week, and sixteen-week marks for follow-up, diet progression, and weigh-ins.

At eight weeks, a new Andrea appeared, looking bright, healthy, happy, and confident. She had lost twenty-one pounds of fat tissue, which gives the appearance of a forty-two-pound weight loss on traditional diets. Her new lab data was markedly improved, with glucose and cholesterol in the normal range. She was exercising by briskly walking forty-five minutes, five times a week. Her clothes were loose and she mentioned that she was hooking her bra two links smaller! She had energy, felt peaceful, and was hopeful.

We advanced her meal plan to Step Two. Andrea was hesitant about adding the required carbohydrate of Step Two because in the past, when she reintroduced carbohydrate in Phase Two of another popular low-carb diet, she regained her weight. I explained that the Miracle is devised specifically for her metabolism and that her fat loss, improved labs, and general well-being would continue. Taking a leap of faith, Andrea moved on to Step Two and returned in a month after losing seven additional pounds of fat (what looks like fourteen pounds on a traditional diet). At this point, Andrea decided to proceed with the Metabolism Miracle and put her gastric bypass plans on the back burner.

Andrea's weight loss continued and, within a year, she had hit her desired weight, with all her labs in the normal range. She lives her life on the maintenance phase of the Miracle, runs five days a week, and plans on entering a five-kilometer run this summer.

SARAH SENDS HER SCALE PACKING

Sarah is a thirty-eight-year-old woman who recently gave birth to her second child, a nine-pound girl, Caroline. She decided to return to her tried-and-true point counting program to drop the pounds she had gained during her pregnancy. Every morning, she dutifully stepped onto her bathroom scale. (Sarah knew just how to stand on the scale to get her lowest weight!) After her previous pregnancy, when she needed to lose weight, her standby diet and exercise program easily did the trick. After Caroline's birth, she told herself, "Within a week, I'll be down about five pounds" (water loss, true, but . . . at least the scale will move!!!) But this time it was different:

Monday morning: 157 pounds . . ."Day 1 of the 'new me'"

Tuesday morning: 157 pounds . . ."I guess it takes a few days to kick in"

Wednesday morning: 158 pounds . . ."Wait a minute, I *gained* weight?"

Thursday morning: 158.5 pounds . . ." This is ridiculous. I'm starving and gaining?"

Friday morning: 156 pounds . . ."Eureka! Progress!"

Saturday morning: 157 pounds . . ."Back to my original weight? The scale must be broken."

Sunday morning: 157.5 pounds . . ."No comment."

Monday morning: 156.5 pounds . . ."Okay, now I'm cooking."

Tuesday morning: 157 pounds . . ."@@#%$! That's it!!!"

Wednesday morning: 157.5 pounds . . ."Diet over!"

After several attempts to lose weight on her original program, Sarah met with me for weight loss. Based on her symptoms, family history, and lab work, she and I discussed her trying the Miracle program. After explaining that her weight loss would always be "different than before," as it was driven by the overmetabolism of carbohydrate, I asked her to wait one month to step on the scale again. She couldn't wait. Every day she stepped on—and sure enough, at first, her weight-loss had no pattern. At the end of one month, though, she had lost appreciable weight and fat, looked great, and felt great. She finally trusted that her body would respond to the program, but in its own way. She now weighs herself monthly and has learned to use her body measurements, clothes size, and energy levels to mark her progress.

THE POWER OF POSITIVE THINKING

In a book that is meant to help you improve your health, lose weight, and enhance well-being, I would be remiss not to include a brief chapter on the power of positive thinking.

Patient after patient walks into my office depressed, frustrated, and exhausted, having lost hope about improving their health and weight. Initially, many have a hard time making eye contact or even smiling. I keep a box of tissues nearby because tears often flow on the first visit. The longer people have lived without help for the symptoms of Metabolism B, the more despondent they feel.

I felt exactly the same way more than twenty-five years ago when my own Metabolism B began to manifest itself and impede my health. I was depressed, lethargic, angry, anxious, and pessimistic. I had difficulty mustering up any good feelings, let alone feeling positive about my future. I had no idea at that time, as type 2 diabetes marched forward in my body, that a hormonal imbalance had shaken up everything in my world, including the way my body used its fuel.

When you start the Metabolism Miracle program, you will learn the simple, straightforward mechanics of how best to eat with your unique metabolism, Metabolism B. I know that parts of this program seem counterintuitive. Who would have thought that you must eat right before bed? It seems wrong to have a snack before you exercise in the morning. And how can a food as healthy as lentil soup bump up your weight more than peanuts or cheese?

I know that you've seen it all when it comes to dieting and you are tired of the disappointments after so much work. But this time around believe that this program, this new understanding of your body and its best maintenance, will change your life in a way that you have long dreamed about. Please take a leap of faith with this program. Part of your job, as you follow the dream, is to believe that it will work.

I never used to believe that one's thoughts could influence the outcome of life. But as I watch my patients' spirits begin to lift on the first eight weeks of the Metabolism Miracle, and see them start to believe again in their power to control their own future, it is like watching a bird that has long been caged take flight. Your body has become your prison, but believing you can change that will help usher you toward a speedy recovery and a bright, healthy future.

I am now a firm believer that your mind, and the thoughts you let it form, very much impact the outcome of every day of your life. If you tell yourself, "It'll never work." "I will never lose this weight." "Why bother?" you may never make it through the first three days of Step One. But when the same people who once looked for fault with everything and everyone, and lived every day feeling miserable and irritable, start to instead tell themselves, "This will work for me." "I will lose this weight and keep it off." "I will know perfect weight and excellent health," they fortify their own conviction and make it all happen with the Miracle.

The more often you tell yourself positive thoughts, the more you will believe the words and feel the positive energy slowly but surely change the way you see the world. Before you fall asleep at night and the very first thing in the morning speak positively to yourself.

Say this . . .	*Instead of this . . .*
"I am getting thinner and healthier every day."	"I don't see anything happening."
"I am doing this very well."	"I hope I can do this."
"I feel so much more alive and energetic."	"I'm tired."
"I am a success."	"I have always failed."
"The Miracle will work for me because it was written for me."	"I hope this works."
"I can feel my energy returning."	"I have no energy."
"My clothes are getting looser every day."	"I look heavy in this outfit."

When you fill your mind and life with positive good thoughts, they will overflow into a positive way of living. *The Metabolism Miracle* starts a new beginning to your life. Expect it to work for you, know it will work for you, and watch it work for you. For the first time in a long time, you will work with your metabolism instead of against it and you will be in tune with your body and newfound health.

PART FOUR
Recipes

BREAKFAST

Easy Egg Cups

For Steps One, Two, and Three; **count as no carb**
Serves 4 (1 egg cup/serving)

> Cooking oil spray
> 4 ounces shredded low-fat cheese
> 8 strips cooked turkey bacon, finely chopped
> 4 whole eggs
> Salt and pepper
> 4 tablespoons light cream
> 4 tablespoons grated Parmesan cheese

Preheat the oven to 350°F. Spray the bottom and sides of 4 cups of a muffin tin with cooking oil spray.

Drop 1 ounce of shredded low-fat cheese into each cup.

Place one-quarter of the chopped turkey bacon in each cup.

Break one egg into each cup, leaving whole.

Add salt and pepper to the cream, mix well, and place 1 tablespoon in each cup.

Sprinkle the top of each cup with 1 tablespoon of grated Parmesan.

Bake for 10 minutes. If desired, brown the cheese under the broiler for 2 to 3 minutes. Serve warm.

MIRACLE QUICHE

For Steps One, Two, and Three; **count as no carb**
Serves 4

> Cooking oil spray
> 1 tablespoon butter
> 1/2 medium onion, diced
> 2 cups sliced mushrooms
> 1 cup diced fresh broccoli florets
> 1/2 cup light cream
> 4 ounces grated low-fat Cheddar cheese
> Salt and pepper
> 6 eggs, beaten

Preheat the oven to 325°F. Spray the bottom and sides of a 9-inch ceramic or glass pie pan with cooking oil spray.

Melt the butter in a skillet and sauté the diced onion, mushrooms, and broccoli until soft.

In a medium saucepan, heat the cream until hot; do not boil. Remove from the heat and stir in the Cheddar cheese until it melts.

Add the sautéed mushrooms, broccoli, salt, and pepper to the melted cheese mixture and let cool for 5 minutes.

Add the beaten eggs to the mixture and mix well.

Pour into the prepared pie pan and bake for 45 to 50 minutes, until the custard is set, or a knife inserted in the center of the quiche comes out clean. Cool on a rack for at least 5 minutes before slicing.

CRUSTLESS HAM, CHEDDAR, AND VEGGIE QUICHE

For Steps One, Two, and Three; **count as no carb**
Serves 4

Cooking oil spray
2 tablespoons butter
2 teaspoons canola oil
1 medium onion, finely chopped
1/2 green bell pepper, seeded and finely chopped
1 cup sliced mushrooms
6 eggs, beaten
1/2 cup light cream
1/4 teaspoon salt
1/8 teaspoon black pepper
1/2 pound ham, diced into small cubes
8 ounces low-fat shredded Cheddar cheese
1 large fresh tomato, seeded and diced
10 ounces frozen chopped spinach, completely thawed with excess
    liquid squeezed out

Preheat the oven to 350°F. Lightly coat a 10-inch pie plate or quiche dish with cooking oil spray and set aside.

In a skillet, melt the butter and oil. Add the chopped onion, green bell pepper, and mushrooms, and sauté until the onions turn glossy and are tender; set this mixture aside.

In the same skillet used for the sautéing, stir together the beaten eggs, light cream, salt, and pepper, and heat for 5 minutes, stirring constantly.

In the bottom of the pie plate, distribute the diced ham, shredded Cheddar cheese, chopped tomato, and spinach. Top with the sautéed vegetable mixture.

Pour the beaten egg mixture over the veggie, ham, and cheese base.

Bake for approximately 50 minutes, or until a knife inserted in the center of the quiche comes out clean. Cool on a rack for at least 5 minutes before slicing.

A Taste of Hot "Cereal"

For Step One, Two, and Three; **count as no carb**
Makes 1/2 cup serving of faux "hot cereal"

 1/4 cup finely chopped almonds
 1/4 cup finely chopped Brazil nuts
 2 tablespoons ground sesame seeds
 1 teaspoon butter
 1/4 cup light cream
 1/8 teaspoon ground cinnamon
 1 (1 g) packet Splenda
 Pinch of salt, if desired

In a food processor, finely process the almonds, Brazil nuts, and sesame seeds.

Place the nut mixture in a microwave-safe cereal bowl.

Add the butter, light cream, cinnamon, Splenda, and salt (if desired) and mix well.

Microwave on high for 30 seconds or until the butter is melted. Stir, close your eyes, and think "hot cereal."

SILVER DOLLAR PANCAKES

For Steps One, Two, and Three (**6 mini pancakes = 5x5 carb food**)

Makes about 30 pancakes; one serving size = 6 pancakes = approximately 3 grams of net carb

> Cooking oil spray
> 1 cup part-skim ricotta cheese
> 1/3 cup soy flour
> 1 tablespoon canola oil
> 1/2 teaspoon vanilla extract
> 1 (1 g) packet Splenda
> Pinch of salt
> 4 eggs, beaten

Spray a griddle pan or skillet with cooking oil spray.

In a mixing bowl, blend together the ricotta cheese, soy flour, canola oil, vanilla, Splenda, and salt.

Fold in the beaten eggs and mix into a batterlike consistency.

Spoon onto the prepared hot pan; lightly brown on both sides.

Serve with carb-free syrup, light whipped cream, or a dollop of carb-free jelly.

APPETIZERS AND SNACKS

CLAM AND CRAB DIP

For Steps One, Two, and Three; **count as no carb**
Makes approximately 2 1/2 cups of dip

   1 (8-ounce) package light cream cheese
   1/4 cup olive oil
   1/4 cup light mayonnaise
   1 (6 1/2-ounce) can minced crabmeat, drained
   1 (6 1/2-ounce) can minced clams, drained
   Salt and pepper
   2 tablespoons finely chopped fresh dill
   1/4 cup finely chopped fresh parsley
   1/4 teaspoon garlic powder
   1/4 teaspoon onion powder
   1 splash hot sauce

In a medium saucepan, over low heat, combine all the ingredients. Stir occasionally for 30 minutes until warmed thoroughly.

Transfer to a covered container and chill overnight.

Serve as a dip for "free veggies"—green or red bell pepper strips or rings, cauliflower or broccoli florets, mushroom caps, whole green beans.

EASY PIZZA

For Steps One, Two, and Three; **count as 5 grams net carb (5x5 carb)**
Serves 1

> Cooking oil spray
> 1 low-carb tortilla or wrap (<5 grams net carb)
> A scant 1/4 cup crushed tomatoes with seasonings
> Salt and pepper
> Dried oregano, basil, onion powder, and/or garlic powder, if desired
> 1/2 cup shredded mozzarella cheese
> Grated Parmesan cheese

Preheat the oven to 350°F. Spray a cookie sheet lightly with cooking spray.

Place the tortilla on the prepared cookie sheet. Spoon the crushed tomatoes evenly over tortilla.

Sprinkle very lightly with salt, pepper, and your favorite pizza spices, such as oregano, garlic powder, onion powder, and/or garlic powder to taste.

Sprinkle evenly with the shredded mozzarella cheese. Top with a sprinkle of Parmesan.

Bake until the cheese thoroughly melts, about 5 minutes

Feta-Stuffed Mushrooms

For Steps One, Two, and Three; **count as no carb**
Serves 2 (1 mushroom per serving)

> Cooking oil spray
> 2 portobello mushrooms (5–6 ounces each)
> Oil from the sun-dried tomatoes (below)
> 1 (4-ounce) package crumbled feta cheese
> 1/2 cup chopped pitted ripe olives
> 2 tablespoons chopped, oil-packed sun-dried tomatoes

Preheat the oven to 425°F. Spray a cookie sheet with cooking oil spray.

Remove and discard the mushroom stems. Place the mushroom caps, stem side up, on the cookie sheet, brush the inside of each mushroom with oil from the sun-dried tomatoes and set aside.

In a small mixing bowl, combine the feta cheese, olives, and sun-dried tomatoes, and mix well.

Divide the cheese mixture equally and place atop the mushrooms.

Bake for 10 minutes until completely heated. Serve warm.

MIRACLE GRILLED CHEESE

For Steps One, Two, and Three; **count as a 5x5 carb**
Serves 1

> Cooking oil spray
> 1 teaspoon butter
> 1 low-carb tortilla or wrap (*with 5 grams or less net carb*)
> 1/2 cup shredded cheese of your choice (light provolone, Cheddar, low-fat American)

In a small nonstick skillet sprayed with cooking oil spray, melt the butter.

Place the tortilla on top of the melted butter; spread the shredded cheese all over the tortilla.

When the tortilla bottom is golden brown and cheese begins to melt, flip the tortilla in half to close it up.

Heat for 15 seconds on both sides. Serve warm.

CRISPY TORTILLA CHIPS

For Steps One, Two, and Three; **count as a 5x5 carb**
Makes 8 tortilla chips, for dipping: 5 grams of net carb/
8 chips per tortilla

> Cooking oil spray
> 1 low-carb tortilla (*with 5 grams or less net carb*)
> Garlic powder
> Salt and pepper
> 1 tablespoon grated Parmesan cheese

Preheat the oven to 425°F. Spray a cookie sheet with cooking oil spray.

Cut the tortilla into eight chip-size triangles. Place the triangles on the cookie sheet.

Lightly spray the tortilla triangles with cooking oil spray.

Immediately sprinkle desired amount of garlic powder, salt, pepper, and Parmesan cheese onto the triangles.

Bake for 5 to 8 minutes, until golden brown and crispy. Watch periodically to make sure they don't burn. Let cool before eating.

Parmesan Chips

For Steps One, Two, and Three; **count as no carb**

> Cooking oil spray
> Coarsely grated Parmesan cheese (from specialty cheese section of grocery stores)

Preheat the oven to 400°F. Spray a cookie sheet with cooking oil spray.

Spoon 1-tablespoon spoonfuls of Parmesan cheese onto the cookie sheet.

Pat down each spoonful to form a little disk.

Bake for 5 minutes. Let cool before you try to remove the chips from the cookie sheet.

SWEET NUT TREAT

For Steps One, Two, and Three; **count as no carb**
Makes 2 cups of sweetened walnut halves

> 2 tablespoons butter
>
> 2 cups walnut halves
>
> 1/2 cup granulated Splenda
>
> 1 tablespoon vanilla extract
>
> 2 tablespoons ground cinnamon
>
> 1/4 teaspoon ground nutmeg

In a large skillet, melt the butter over medium heat; when the butter is melted, add the nuts and stir and coat with the butter.

Sprinkle with the Splenda, vanilla, cinnamon, and nutmeg, and stir well to coat the nuts.

Remove from the skillet, lay flat on a dish, and allow to cool. Store in an airtight container.

Ham and Cream Cheese "Packets"

For Steps One, Two, and Three; **count as no carb**

Makes approximately 16 "package" appetizers

> 4 ounces (half of an 8-ounce package) light cream cheese, softened
> 1/4 cup finely chopped scallions
> 1/2 teaspoon prepared horseradish, if desired
> Salt and pepper, if desired
> 1 pound sliced deli ham (16 slices)
> Approximately 16 tiny pitted olives, for garnish

In a small mixing bowl, mix the softened cream cheese, scallions, horseradish, salt, and pepper.

Place a spoonful of the cream cheese mixture in center of each piece of ham.

Make a square of each ham slice by folding in the sides toward the middle.

Top the little "packet" with an olive and secure with a toothpick.

SUN-DRIED TOMATO DIP

For Steps One, Two, and Three; **count as no carb**
Makes about 2 1/2 cups of dip

  8 ounces low-fat cottage cheese
  8 ounces ricotta cheese
  1 finely chopped green onion
  1/2 cup finely chopped red or green bell pepper
  1/4 cup finely chopped oil-packed sun-dried tomatoes
  1 tablespoon fresh basil, or 1 teaspoon dried
  1 teaspoon lemon juice
  1/8 teaspoon salt
  1/8 teaspoon black pepper

Combine all ingredients in blender or food processor. Blend until smooth. Refrigerate for at least 2 hours.

Serve as a dip for "free veggies"—bell pepper rings, broccoli florets, celery sticks, or mushroom caps.

SOUPS AND SALADS

Cabbage Salad

For Steps One, Two, and Three; **count as no carb**
Serves 6 to 8

   1 medium head cabbage, finely chopped
   1 cup light sour cream
   2 tablespoons finely chopped fresh parsley
   1/3 cup olive oil
   1/3 cup light mayonnaise
   2 tablespoons white vinegar
   1/4 teaspoon onion powder
   Salt and pepper

In a large mixing bowl, combine the cabbage, sour cream, and parsley. Distribute the sour cream over the cabbage thoroughly.

In a small bowl, whisk together the oil, mayonnaise, vinegar, onion powder, salt, and pepper.

Pour the dressing over the cabbage and toss.

Cover and chill before serving.

Miracle "Potato-less" Soup

For Steps One, Two, and Three; **count as no carb**
Serves 6

> 1 head cauliflower, broken into tiny florets
> 2 finely chopped scallions
> 1 teaspoon finely chopped garlic
> 4 cups chicken broth (can be low-sodium if desired)
> 4 ounces light sour cream
> 4 ounces shredded light Cheddar cheese
> 1/4 cup butter
> 6 strips turkey bacon, microwaved until crisp and finely chopped
> Salt and pepper

Gently boil the cauliflower florets, chopped scallions, and garlic in the chicken broth. After 10 to 15 minutes, check for complete tenderness of the cauliflower.

Microwave the turkey bacon on high setting, on paper toweling, for 3 to 5 minutes, until crisp.

Remove the cauliflower from the broth, reserving the broth, and place in a mixing bowl or food processor.

Add the sour cream, shredded Cheddar cheese, and butter to the cauliflower and mix (use a hand mixer or food processor) until smooth.

Return this mixture to the broth. Add the finely chopped bacon and stir over medium heat. Additional chicken broth may be added at this time for a thinner soup.

Add salt and pepper to taste.

CORN BISQUE

For Steps Two and Three; **1 cup = 1 carb serving**
Serves 4

2 teaspoons olive oil

2 finely chopped tablespoons scallions

1/2 cup diced onion

1/4 cup diced celery

2 tablespoons whole wheat flour

2 cups frozen corn kernels

1 1/2 cups chicken broth

1/2 teaspoon Worcestershire sauce

1 drop hot sauce (optional)

1/2 teaspoon dried dill

1/2 teaspoon pepper

1/2 cup light cream

In a medium saucepan, heat the olive oil on medium-high heat.

Add the scallions, onion, and celery, and stir constantly until the onion is soft and translucent.

Sprinkle the flour over the cooked veggies and stir for about 2 minutes.

Add all the remaining ingredients except the cream and heat for 10 minutes. Allow to cool slightly.

Transfer two-thirds of the veggie mixture into a blender and puree until smooth.

Add this puree to the remaining mixture and stir in the cream.

Serve warm.

ITALIAN VEGETABLE SOUP

For Steps Two and Three; **1 cup = 1 carb serving**
Serves 6 to 8

Cooking oil spray

1 pound ground mild Italian sausage, ground turkey sausage, or
   lean ground beef

1 cup diced onion

1 cup sliced celery

1 cup sliced carrots

1 (15-ounce) can red kidney beans, drained

1 (15-ounce) can black beans, drained

2 cups beef broth

1/4 cup finely chopped fresh parsley

2 (16-ounce) cans diced tomatoes

1/2 teaspoon salt

1/4 teaspoon oregano

1/4 teaspoon basil

1/4 teaspoon black pepper

2 cups shredded cabbage

Parmesan cheese, if desired

In a large skillet coated with cooking oil spray, brown the meat and drain.

Add all the ingredients except the cabbage and cheese, and bring to a boil.

Lower the heat, partially cover, and simmer for 30 minutes.

Add the cabbage and simmer for another 15 minutes.

Add Parmesan cheese to individual servings, if desired.

SWEET-AND-SOUR CUKES

For Steps One, Two, and Three; **count as no carb**
Serves 6

>   2 cups sliced, unpeeled well-washed cucumbers
>   1 cup very thinly sliced red onion
>   1/4 cup white vinegar
>   1/4 teaspoon dried dill
>   1 tablespoon powdered Splenda
>   Salt and pepper

Place the sliced cucumber in a medium mixing bowl and add the onion.

In a small mixing bowl, whisk together the vinegar, dill, Splenda, salt, and pepper to taste.

Pour the sauce over the cukes and chill for at least 1 hour.

Toss before serving. Serve chilled.

TENDER SPINACH SALAD

For Steps One, Two, and Three; **count as no carb**
Serves 4

> 10 ounces fresh baby spinach, washed and dried
> 1 cup fresh mushroom slices
> 4 hard-cooked eggs, chopped
> 12 slices turkey bacon, cooked and chopped
> 1/2 cup olive oil
> 1/2 cup sour cream
> 1/4 cup red wine vinegar
> 1/2 teaspoon dry mustard
> Salt and pepper

In a large bowl, toss the spinach, mushrooms, eggs, and cooked bacon.

In a separate mixing bowl, whisk together the olive oil, sour cream, vinegar, mustard, salt, and pepper to taste.

Add the dressing to the veggies and toss to coat.

POTATO-ISH SALAD

For Steps One, Two, and Three; **count as no carb**
Serves 4 to 6

> 1 head cauliflower, broken into small florets
> 1/2 cup light mayonnaise
> 1/2 cup light cream
> 1/4 teaspoon mustard (spicy preferred)
> 1/4 teaspoon celery seeds
> 1 teaspoon powdered Splenda
> 1/2 onion, very finely chopped
> 1/2 green bell pepper, very finely chopped
> 2 hard-cooked eggs, diced, if desired
> Salt and pepper

Cook the cauliflower in a large pot of boiling, salted water. Check for tenderness after 10 minutes. The cauliflower should be very soft, the texture of cooked potatoes for potato salad.

Drain and pat dry.

In a large mixing bowl, whisk together the mayo, cream, mustard, celery seed, and Splenda.

Add the cauliflower, onion, peppers, and diced egg to the dressing and toss lightly to coat the cauliflower.

Add salt and pepper to taste. This salad tastes best after at least 3 hours of refrigeration.

COLD PEA SALAD

For Steps Two and Three; **2/3 cup = 1 carb serving**
Serves 4

> 2 cups frozen peas, thawed and dried
> 1/2 cup light sour cream
> 1/2 cup plain yogurt
> 3/4 cup chopped scallions
> Salt and pepper

Place the peas in a bowl.

In a medium mixing bowl, whisk the sour cream, yogurt, scallions, salt, and pepper to taste.

Pour the dressing over the peas and mix well. Cover and refrigerate until cold.

Serve chilled.

Pasta Primavera Salad

For Steps Two and Three; **1 cup = 1 carb serving**
Serves 8

- 1 cup diced carrots
- 1 cup diced yellow squash
- 1 cup diced red onion
- 1 cup small cauliflower florets
- 1 cup small broccoli florets
- 1 cup light ranch dressing
- 2 cups cooked (1/2 pound dried) whole wheat pasta shapes (al dente recommended)
- 1/2 cup grated Parmesan cheese
- 1 cup diced fresh tomato

Steam all the veggies except the tomato until crisp-tender.

Transfer to a large mixing bowl, mix with the ranch dressing, and marinate for several hours in the refrigerator.

Mix the marinated veggies with the cooked pasta, until well coated.

Add grated Parmesan and the diced tomato, and mix thoroughly.

Serve chilled.

Three-Bean Salad

For Steps Two and Three; **1/2 cup = 1 carb serving**
Makes 10 servings

> 1 (14-ounce) can cut green beans, drained
>
> 1 (14-ounce) can kidney beans, drained
>
> 1 (14-ounce) can chickpeas (garbanzo beans), drained
>
> 1 medium red onion, finely chopped
>
> 1/2 cup white vinegar
>
> 1/4 cup olive oil
>
> 3 tablespoons powdered Splenda
>
> 1/4 teaspoon salt
>
> 1/4 teaspoon pepper

In a large mixing bowl, combine the three types of drained beans and the onions and mix well.

In a small mixing bowl, whisk together the vinegar, olive oil, Splenda, salt, and pepper.

Pour the dressing over the beans and mix.

Refrigerate for at least 2 hours before serving.

ENTRÉES

Cheesy Burgers

For Steps One, Two, and Three; **count no carb**
Serves 5

> 1 pound lean ground beef or lean ground turkey
> 1/4 pound ground turkey sausage
> 2 cloves garlic, finely chopped
> 1/2 medium onion, finely chopped
> 2 eggs, beaten
> Salt and pepper
> 1 1/2 cups shredded Cheddar cheese

In a large mixing bowl, combine all ingredients except the Cheddar. Wearing plastic gloves, hand mix the ingredients well.

Form into ten very thin patties (half the size of your normal pre-cooked burger).

Place 1/4 cup of shredded cheese between two patties and seal so the meat is entirely enclosing the cheese. Repeat with the remaining meat mixture and cheese.

Grill on an outdoor or indoor countertop grill, or broil, until cooked to individual preference.

BROILED TURKEY BURGERS

For Steps One, Two, and Three; **count as no carb**
Serves 4

> Cooking oil spray
> 2 tablespoons olive oil
> 1/2 cup finely chopped green bell pepper
> 1/2 cup finely chopped celery
> 1 clove garlic, minced
> 1/2 cup finely chopped onion
> 1 pound ground turkey
> 2 eggs, beaten
> 1 teaspoon prepared mustard
> Salt and pepper

Preheat the broiler. Coat a broiler pan with nonstick cooking spray.

Spray a large nonstick skillet with cooking oil spray and place over medium-high heat.

Heat the olive oil in the pan and add the green pepper, celery, garlic, and onion. Sauté for about 5 minutes. Set aside to cool.

In a medium mixing bowl, combine the sautéed veggies, ground turkey, eggs, mustard, salt, and pepper. Mix together until well combined. Shape into four patties.

Put the patties on the prepared broiler pan and broil for about 5 minutes per side.

Steps Two and Three: Serve on an 11–20 gram net carb bun = 1 carb serving.

CHICKEN PAPRIKASH

For Steps One, Two, and Three; **count as no carb**
Serves 4 to 6

    1/4 cup olive oil
    2 cloves garlic, sliced
    3 pounds skinless chicken parts (legs, thighs, breast)
    Salt and pepper
    1 small green bell pepper, chopped
    2 tablespoons paprika
    1 cup chicken broth, plus extra as needed for desired consistency
    1/2 teaspoon onion powder
    8 ounces mushroom caps or sliced mushrooms
    1 cup light sour cream

Heat the olive oil and sliced garlic in a large saucepan over medium heat until the garlic browns. Remove and discard the garlic.

Sprinkle the chicken with salt and pepper on both sides.

Add the chicken, green pepper, paprika, onion powder, and chicken broth, and onion powder to the saucepan and cook for 30 minutes over low heat.

Add the mushrooms. Continue to cook until the chicken is tender, about 15 more minutes, adding chicken broth as needed to maintain the level of liquid during the cooking process.

Transfer the cooked chicken pieces to a platter.

Stir the sour cream into the saucepan that the chicken was cooked in and add enough chicken broth to make a gravylike consistency.

Pour the gravy over the chicken and serve hot.

Chunky Chicken Salad

For Steps One, Two, and Three; **count as no carb**
Serves 4

> 1/2 cup light sour cream
> 1/2 cup light mayonnaise
> 2 tablespoons fresh lemon juice
> 1/2 teaspoon salt
> 1/4 teaspoon black pepper
> 2 cups cooked and cubed boneless, skinless chicken breast
> 1/2 green bell pepper, chopped
> 1 small red onion, chopped
> 1/4 cup finely chopped fresh dill
> 1/4 cup finely chopped fresh parsley
> 1/2 cup pitted, sliced black olives

In a medium mixing bowl, combine the sour cream, mayonnaise, lemon juice, salt, and pepper. Blend well.

Add the cubed chicken, green pepper, onion, dill, parsley, and olives. Mix well.

Refrigerate for at least 1 hour prior to serving.

Miracle "Spaghetti"

For Steps One, Two, and Three; **count as no carb**
Serves 4 to 6

  1 spaghetti squash
  Cooking oil spray
  1 pound lean ground turkey or lean ground beef
  2 cloves garlic, minced
  1/2 cup chopped onion
  1/2 cup chopped green bell pepper
  2 (14-ounce) cans crushed tomatoes with basil and herbs
  1/2 cup white wine
  1 cup grated Parmesan cheese

Cut the spaghetti squash in half and remove the seeds.

Place, face down, in microwave-safe dish with a 1/2-inch depth of water on the bottom.

Cover with plastic wrap. Make a few slits in the plastic wrap for ventilation.

Microwave on high until tender, 20 to 30 minutes.

Over medium heat, in a large skillet sprayed with cooking oil spray, brown the ground turkey, garlic, onion, and green pepper for about 10 minutes, until the meat is cooked.

When the meat is cooked, add the crushed tomatoes and wine, and simmer for about 30 minutes.

After the squash is cooked and has cooled enough to handle, use a fork to pull/shred it into a large bowl. It will actually look like strands of spaghetti!

Divide the spaghetti among four to six plates, top with the meat sauce, and sprinkle with Parmesan.

PHILLY STEAK AND CHEESE

For Steps One, Two, and Three; **count as no carb**
Serves 4

> Cooking oil spray
> 1 pound "minute"/wafer steaks (beef or chicken)
> 2 green bell peppers, cored and sliced in 1-inch slices
> 1 large onion, diced
> 2 cloves garlic, finely chopped
> 1/2 cup beef or chicken broth
> 1 cup shredded provolone cheese

Preheat the oven to 350°F. Spray a large skillet and a shallow baking pan with cooking oil spray.

Break the steaks into quarters and quickly brown in the skillet. Drain off the excess fat and place the browned steak quarters in the baking pan.

In the hot skillet, over medium-high heat, sauté the pepper, onion, and garlic until golden brown. Spoon the sautéed veggies on top of the steak.

Pour the broth over the steak and veggies.

Bake, uncovered, for 20 minutes.

Top with shredded provolone cheese and broil for 3 minutes, until the cheese gets bubbly.

Step One: Serve inside a low-carb wrap (<5 grams of net carb) = 5x5 carb.

Steps Two and Three: Serve in a warm, 11–20 gram net carb bun = 1 carb serving.

SEAFOOD DELIGHT

For Steps One, Two, and Three; **count as no carb**
Serves 4 to 6

1/4 cup butter
1/4 cup olive oil
1/4 cup white wine
2 teaspoons crushed garlic
Cooking oil spray
1/2 pound flounder filet
1 pound large sea scallops
1 pound whole jumbo shrimp
2 tablespoons finely chopped fresh parsley
1/4 cup grated Parmesan cheese

Preheat the oven to 400° F.

In a small saucepan over medium heat, melt the butter, then add the olive oil, white wine, and crushed garlic. Heat until the garlic is lightly browned, then remove and discard the garlic. Set the sauce aside.

Spray a glass baking dish with cooking oil spray. Cut the flounder into six pieces. Arrange the flounder, scallops, and shrimp in the baking dish.

Pour the sauce over the fish and sprinkle with the chopped parsley. Bake, uncovered, until the fish is flaky and thoroughly cooked. Sprinkle with grated Parmesan cheese, if desired, and serve.

SHISH KEBAB

For Steps One, Two, and Three; **count as no carb**
Serves 4 to 6

  1/4 cup olive oil
  1/2 cup Italian dressing
  2 tablespoons lemon juice
  3 large cloves garlic, crushed
  1/4 cup white wine
  1/4 teaspoon salt
  1/4 teaspoon pepper
  1/4 teaspoon dried oregano
  1/4 teaspoon dried rosemary
  1 1/2 pounds leg of lamb, or London broil, cubed for kebabs
  1 large green bell pepper, seeded and cut into 8 chunks
  1 large red bell pepper, seeded and cut into 8 chunks
  1 large red onion, cut into 8 chunks
  12 medium mushroom caps

In medium mixing bowl, combine the olive oil, Italian dressing, lemon juice, garlic, wine, and seasonings.

Pour the marinade over the lamb cubes and stir to completely coat the lamb. Cover tightly and refrigerate for 24 hours, occasionally stirring the sauce over the lamb.

The next day, preheat the broiler.

Remove the lamb cubes from the marinade (reserve the marinade) and thread on skewers to contain only lamb. Other skewers should be used separately to create pepper kebabs, onion kebabs, and mushroom kebabs, as they will all be grilled for different amounts of time.

Place the shish kebabs on a broiling tray. Baste all with the marinade.

Broil about 6 inches from the heat source: the lamb skewers for 10 minutes, the pepper and the onion skewers for 4 minutes, and the mushroom skewers for 3 minutes.

Remove the meat and veggies from the skewers and set aside to cool enough to be handled.

Rethread a skewer with a cube of cooked lamb, then a piece of pepper, then a piece of onion, then a mushroom, and repeat until all ingredients have been used on as many skewers as will hold them.

Baste all the shish kebabs with the marinade.

Return the skewers to the broiler, turning frequently, until the meat is totally cooked. (Safety note: Because the marinade has been used for raw meat, be sure to cook through at high heat before serving.)

SWEDISH MEATBALLS

For Steps One, Two, and Three; **count as no carb**
Serves 4; 7 meatballs/serving

> 1 pound lean ground beef
> 1 medium onion, finely chopped
> 1 medium green bell pepper, seeded and finely chopped
> 2 cloves garlic, finely chopped
> 1/4 cup finely chopped fresh dill
> 1/4 cup finely chopped fresh parsley
> 1/2 teaspoon Italian seasoning
> 1/4 teaspoon grated nutmeg
> 1 teaspoon dried dill
> 1 large egg, beaten
> 1/2 teaspoon salt
> Black pepper
> Cooking oil spray
> 2 tablespoons olive oil
> 3/4 cup beef broth
> 1/4 cup white wine

In a large mixing bowl, combine the ground beef, onion, green pepper, garlic, dill, parsley, spices, beaten egg, salt, and pepper.

Using plastic gloves, use your hands to mix the ingredients evenly. Form into about thirty 1-inch mini meatballs.

Spray a nonstick skillet with cooking spray and add the 2 tablespoons of olive oil. Cook over medium heat.

Cook the meatballs, in batches if necessary, shaking the skillet occasionally, until they are browned on all sides and cooked through.

Remove the meatballs from the skillet and place on paper toweling, to drain excess grease.

Add the beef broth and wine to the skillet and cover. Turn up the heat and cook over high heat for about 3 minutes.

Add the meatballs back to the pan and cook in the sauce for 10 minutes, spooning the sauce over the meatballs as it thickens.

Serve immediately.

Slow-Cooked Beef and Bean Chili

For Steps Two and Three; **count as 1 cup = 1 carb serving**
Serves 8

> 1 (14-ounce) can diced tomatoes, undrained
>
> 1 (14-ounce) can chopped tomatoes and green chile peppers,
>   undrained
>
> 1 cup vegetable juice cocktail or tomato juice
>
> 1 cup beef broth
>
> 1 tablespoon chile powder
>
> 1 teaspoon ground cumin
>
> 1 teaspoon dried oregano
>
> 3 cloves garlic, peeled and minced
>
> 2 pounds boneless beef chuck roast, cut into 1-inch cubes
>
> 2 large onions, chopped
>
> 3 stalks celery, chopped
>
> 1 large green bell pepper, seeded and chopped
>
> 1 (15-ounce can) kidney beans, drained
>
> 1 (15-ounce can) chickpeas (garbanzo beans), drained

In a 6-quart slow cooker (such as a Crock Pot), combine diced and chopped tomatoes, vegetable juice, beef broth, chile powder, cumin, oregano, garlic, beef, onions, celery, and green pepper.

Cover and cook on the low heat setting for 8 to 10 hours, or high heat setting for 4 to 5 hours.

Stir in the kidney beans and chickpeas.

Cook on the high setting for 15 minutes longer.

Eggplant Rollatini

For Steps One, Two, and Three; **count as no carb**
Serves 6

> 3 medium eggplants, cut lengthwise into 1/4-inch slices
> Salt
> Coking oil spray
> Olive oil
> 2 cups part-skim ricotta cheese
> 1 large egg, beaten
> 1 cup shredded mozzarella cheese
> 1/2 cup grated Parmesan cheese
> 1/4 cup finely chopped fresh parsley
> 2 cups seasoned crushed tomatoes or your own marinara sauce,
>   made without added tomato paste or tomato sauce

Preheat the oven to 350°F.

Lightly sprinkle both sides of the sliced eggplant with salt. Place the eggplant slices in a colander in the sink for about 15 minutes. Rinse and blot dry the eggplant slices.

Over medium heat, heat a large sauté pan sprayed with cooking oil spray. Add about 2 tablespoons of olive oil.

Add the eggplant in batches and cook until soft and pliable, replacing the olive oil as needed. Transfer the eggplant to a platter.

In a large mixing bowl, mix the ricotta, egg, mozzarella, Parmesan, and parsley.

One eggplant slice at a time, spread the cheese mixture over an entire slice and then roll up. Spray a glass baking dish with cooking oil spray. Place the roll, seam side down, in the glass baking dish.

After all the eggplant is rolled, pour the marinara over the rolls and top with a little more Parmesan, if desired.

Bake for 30 minutes and serve.

PASTA-FREE VEGGIE LASAGNE

For Steps One, Two, and Three; **count one 4 by 4-inch**
serving as no carb
Makes 12 servings

Cooking oil spray

1 large or two small eggplants, cut lengthwise into 1/2-inch slices

2 pounds part-skim ricotta cheese

4 cloves garlic, chopped

1/4 cup grated Parmesan cheese

2 cups shredded part-skim mozzarella (reserve 1/2 cup for the top
   layer)

1 bunch fresh basil, chopped

1 tablespoon dried Italian seasoning

Salt and pepper

1 small onion, chopped

1 medium bell pepper (red, yellow, or orange), seeded and chopped

4 cups sliced mushrooms

1 bunch broccoli, florets only, coarsely chopped

3 ounces fresh spinach, chopped

2 cups crushed tomatoes, or your own marinara recipe, made with
   no added tomato paste or tomato sauce

3 small zucchini, cut lengthwise into 1/8-inch slices

3 small yellow squash, cut lengthwise into 1/8-inch slices

Preheat the oven to 350°F. Spray a baking sheet with cooking oil
spray.

Arrange the eggplant slices on the baking sheet and bake for 15 to
20 minutes, until flexible but not completely cooked.

In a mixing bowl, mix the ricotta with half of the chopped garlic.
Stir in the Parmesan and 1 1/2 cups of the mozzarella cheese,
chopped basil, Italian seasoning, salt, and pepper, and set aside.

Sauté the onion, remaining chopped garlic, pepper, mushrooms, and broccoli for about 5 minutes. Add the chopped spinach and remove from the heat. Allow to cool and then add to the ricotta mixture.

To assemble, spread a thin layer of the crushed tomatoes in a large baking dish, such as a 3-quart Pyrex lasagne dish, then layer:

Eggplant slices
Ricotta mixture
Zucchini or squash slices
Crushed tomatoes
Eggplant slices
Ricotta mixture
Zucchini or squash slices
Crushed tomatoes
Ricotta mixture, and so on

Layer until you run out of ingredients! End with a layer of zucchini or eggplant and top with crushed tomatoes or your sauce. Sprinkle with the reserved 1/2 cup of mozzarella.

Bake for 1 to 1 1/2 hours, until hot and bubbly.

Slow-Cooked Lamb with Wild Rice

For Steps Two and Three; **1 cup = 1 carb serving**
Serves 6

>   Cooking oil spray
>   2 pounds boneless lamb shoulder roast
>   2 tablespoons olive oil
>   1 cup vegetable or tomato juice
>   1 1/2 cups beef broth
>   1 cup uncooked wild rice
>   1 teaspoon curry powder
>   1/2 teaspoon salt
>   2 medium carrots, diced
>   2 stalks celery, diced
>   1 small onion, diced
>   Salt and pepper

Have ready a 4-quart slow cooker.

In a large nonstick skillet coated with cooking spray, brown the meat on all sides in the 2 tablespoons of olive oil.

In the slow cooker, combine the vegetable juice, beef broth, wild rice, curry powder, salt, carrots, celery, onions, salt, and pepper.

Place the roast in the cooker.

Cover and cook on the low heat setting for 8 to 9 hours, or on the high heat setting for 4 to 4 1/2 hours.

STUFFED PEPPERS

For Steps Two and Three; **1 stuffed pepper = 1 carb serving**
Makes 4 servings

> 4 medium green bell peppers
> 1/2 cup sugar-free ketchup
> 1 cup water
> 1 teaspoon Worcestershire sauce
> 1/2 pound ground turkey sausage
> 1 cup cooked brown rice
> 1 large egg, beaten
> 1 cup frozen corn
> 1 teaspoon salt
> 1/4 teaspoon pepper
> Cooking oil spray

Preheat the oven to 350°F.

Wash the peppers, cut the tops off (reserve the tops), core and remove seeds, and set aside.

In a small mixing bowl, whisk together the ketchup, water, and Worcestershire sauce, and set aside.

In a large mixing bowl, mix together the sausage, rice, egg, corn, salt, and pepper.

Put one-quarter of the mixture in each pepper. Replace the top of each pepper.

Spray a baking dish with cooking oil spray and place the filled peppers in the dish. Pour the ketchup mixture over the stuffed peppers.

Bake for 45 minutes.

SIDE DISHES

BROCCOLI-CHEESE CASSEROLE

For Steps One, Two, and Three; **count as no carb**
Serves 4

  2 cups reduced-fat shredded Cheddar cheese
  2 cups sliced mushrooms
  1 cup chopped scallions
  1/2 cup light cream
  1/4 cup olive oil
  1/2 teaspoon salt
  2 cups chopped fresh broccoli
  Cooking oil spray

Preheat the oven to 350°F.

In a medium saucepan over low heat, combine all the ingredients. Cook for 5 minutes, stirring constantly.

Coat a 2-quart casserole dish with cooking oil spray. When the cheese melts, spoon the mixture into the casserole.

Bake for 30 minutes.

Serve warm.

MASHED CAULIFLOWER

For Steps One, Two, and Three; **count as no carb**
Serves 4

> 1 head cauliflower, florets only
> 2 cloves garlic, finely chopped
> 1 (14-ounce) can chicken broth
> 1/2 teaspoon salt
> 1/4 teaspoon pepper
> 1 tablespoon butter
> 1/4 cup light sour cream
> 1/2 cup reduced-fat shredded Cheddar cheese
> Salt and pepper

In a medium saucepan over medium high heat, bring the cauliflower, garlic, broth, and salt to a boil.

Reduce the heat to medium and simmer until extremely tender. Drain, reserving the broth.

Place the cauliflower in a blender with the pepper, butter, sour cream, and Cheddar. Puree, adding broth as needed for a mashed-potato consistency. Salt and pepper to taste.

Serve warm as you would mashed potatoes.

ZUCCHINI AND ONIONS

For Steps One, Two, and Three; **count as no carb**
Serves 4

    Cooking oil spray
    1 tablespoon olive oil
    3 large zucchini, peeled and cut into 1/2-inch slices
    1 medium onion, finely chopped
    1/2 cup chopped walnuts
    1/4 teaspoon grated nutmeg
    1/4 teaspoon dried dill
    Salt and pepper

In a large skillet sprayed with cooking oil spray, heat the olive oil over medium heat.

Add the sliced zucchini and onions and cook, stirring occasionally, for 10 minutes, until tender.

Add the walnuts, nutmeg, dill, salt, and pepper to taste.

Stir and cook for an additional minute.

Serve warm.

SWEET POTATO FRIES

For Steps Two and Three; **eight 1/4-inch fries = 1 carb serving**

Serves 4

Cooking oil spray (for pan)

2 sweet potatoes, peeled and cut lengthwise in 1/4-inch strips

Olive oil cooking spay (for potatoes)

Salt and pepper

1 teaspoon ground cinnamon

2 tablespoons powdered Splenda

Preheat the oven to 450°F. Coat a cookie sheet with cooking oil spray.

Arrange the sweet potatoes strips on the sheet. Do not overlap.

Spray the potatoes with the olive oil cooking spray and sprinkle with salt and pepper.

Bake, turning every 10 minutes, for 30 to 45 minutes, or until tender.

When done, sprinkle with cinnamon and Splenda.

Serve warm.

TABBOULEH

For Steps Two and Three; **1/2 cup = 1 carb serving**
Makes 6 servings

> 1 cup uncooked bulgur
> 2 cups boiling water
> 1/3 cup lemon juice
> 1/2 teaspoon salt
> 1/4 teaspoon black pepper
> 2 garlic cloves, minced
> 3 medium tomatoes, seeded and chopped
> 1 cup finely chopped parsley
> 1 cup finely chopped scallions
> 1/2 cup finely chopped mint leaves

Combine the bulgur and boiling water in a bowl and let soak for 1 hour.

In a large mixing bowl, combine the lemon juice, salt, pepper, and garlic.

Drain the bulgur and add to the lemon juice mixture. Add the other ingredients and mix thoroughly.

Cover tightly and refrigerate for at least 1 hour.

Serve chilled.

BAKED TREATS AND OTHER SWEETS

BAKED APPLES

For Steps Two and Three; **1 filled apple = 1 carb serving**
Serves 4

> Cooking oil spray
> 4 tablespoons butter, softened
> 4 tablespoons powdered Splenda
> 1/2 teaspoon ground cinnamon
> 1/2 teaspoon grated nutmeg
> 1/2 teaspoon ground allspice
> 4 large baking apples (such as Empire, Cortland, Golden Delicious, Winesap), washed and cored

Preheat the oven to 350°F. Coat a baking dish with cooking oil spray.

In a small mixing bowl, blend the butter, Splenda, and spices.
Divide evenly and spoon inside the apples.
Place the filled apples in baking dish coated with cooking oil spray.
Bake for 30 minutes, or until the apples are tender.
Serve warm.

CHOCOLATE BROWNIE MUFFINS

For Steps One, Two, and Three; **1 muffin = 5x5 carb**
Makes 20 to 24 muffins

> 5 ounces unsweetened baking chocolate
>
> 2 cups powdered Splenda
>
> 1 3/4 cups soy flour
>
> 1 1/2 teaspoons baking powder
>
> 1 1/2 teaspoons baking soda
>
> 1 teaspoon salt
>
> 2 eggs
>
> 1 (16-ounce container) light sour cream (or use just 8 ounces for a
>   less moist muffin)
>
> 1/2 cup canola oil
>
> 2 teaspoons vanilla extract
>
> 1 cup boiling water
>
> 1/2 cup finely chopped walnuts, if desired

Preheat the oven to 350°F.

Line 20 to 24 muffin cups with cupcake liners.

Microwave the unsweetened chocolate on high for about 2 minutes, until it melts. Cover while microwaving to avoid spattering.

Combine the dry ingredients in a mixing bowl.

Add the eggs, melted chocolate, sour cream, oil, and vanilla. Stir in the nuts.

Slowly add the boiling water while mixing to a smooth batter. The batter will be thin.

Fill each muffin cup two-thirds full.

Bake for 22 to 25 minutes.

Cool on cooling rack.

These muffins are great for freezing in freezer bags and pulling out as needed. They can be topped with light whipped cream. This is a 5x5 carb, so wait 5 hours before having another 5x5 carb.

"GUILDED" CINNAMON MUFFINS

For Step One, Two, and Three; **each muffin = 5x5 carb**
Makes 24 muffins

4 cups soy flour

1 1/2 teaspoons baking soda

1 1/2 teaspoons baking powder

1 teaspoon salt

5 teaspoons ground cinnamon

4 eggs

1/2 cup canola oil

1 1/2 cups granulated Splenda

1 (16-ounce) container light sour cream

Preheat the oven to 350°F.

Coat 24 muffin cups with cooking oil spray or line with cupcake liners.

Mix together the soy flour, baking soda, baking powder, salt, and cinnamon in a large mixing bowl.

In a separate bowl, beat the eggs and blend with the oil and Splenda. Mix together for about 30 seconds.

Add the egg mixture to the dry mixture and blend in the sour cream.

Pour the batter into the prepared muffin cups.

Bake for 25 minutes, or until lightly browned.

Cool on a cooling rack.

ZUCCHINI MUFFINS

For Steps One, Two, and Three; **1 muffin = 5x5 carb**
Makes 20 to 24 muffins

> 4 cups soy flour
> 1/3 cup ground flaxseed
> 1 1/2 teaspoons baking soda
> 1 1/2 teaspoons baking powder
> 1 teaspoon salt
> 1 1/2 teaspoons ground cinnamon
> 4 eggs
> 3/4 cup vegetable oil (could be 1/2 cup)
> 1 1/2 cups sugar substitute, such as Splenda (could be less to taste)
> 2 medium zucchini, shredded (about 2 cups)
> 1 cup light sour cream
> 1 cup walnut pieces (optional)

Preheat the oven to 350°F.

Coat 24 muffin cups with cooking oil spray or line with cupcake liners.

Whisk together the soy flour, ground flaxseed, baking soda, baking powder, salt, and cinnamon in a large bowl.

In a separate bowl, mix the eggs, oil, and sugar substitute for 30 seconds, until the sugar substitute is dissolved. Stir in the shredded zucchini.

Stir the egg mixture into the flour mixture. Stir in the sour cream and then the walnuts, if using. Pour the batter into the prepared muffin pan, filling the cups three-quarters full. If all 24 cups will not be used, fill the empty cups with a few tablespoons of water.

Bake for 23 to 25 minutes, or until crowned and lightly browned.

Cinnamon Ricotta Pudding

For Steps One, Two, and Three; **count as no carb**

Serves 1

  1/2 cup part-skim ricotta cheese
  1 tablespoon low-fat sour cream
  1/4 teaspoon vanilla extract
  1/4 teaspoon ground cinnamon
  1 (1 g) packet Splenda
  Light whipped cream

Mix together the ricotta, sour cream, vanilla extract, cinnamon, and Splenda in a dessert bowl. Chill and top with light whipped cream before serving.

CHOCOLATE RICOTTA PUDDING

For Steps One, Two, and Three; **count as no carb**
Serves 1

>   1/2 cup part-skim ricotta cheese
>   1 tablespoon low-fat sour cream
>   1/2 teaspoon unsweetened cocoa powder
>   1/4 teaspoon vanilla extract
>   1 (1 g) packet Splenda
>   Light whipped cream

Mix together the ricotta, sour cream, cocoa powder, vanilla extract, and Splenda in a dessert bowl. Chill and top with light whipped cream before serving.

LEMON RICOTTA PUDDING

For Steps One, Two, and Three; **count as no carb**

Serves 1

> 1/2 cup part-skim ricotta cheese
>
> 1 tablespoon low-fat sour cream
>
> 1/4 teaspoon grated lemon zest
>
> 1/4 teaspoon vanilla extract
>
> 1 (1 g) packet Splenda
>
> Light whipped cream

Mix together the ricotta, sour cream, lemon zest, vanilla extract, and Splenda in a dessert bowl. Chill and top with light whipped cream before serving.

COOL AND CREAMY GELATIN MOUSSE

For Steps One, Two, and Three; **count as no carb**
Makes about eight 1/2-cup servings

1 (4-serving) package sugar-free Jell-O, your choice of flavor
1 (8-ounce) container light cream cheese, softened
1/2 cup light sour cream
1 cup light whipping cream
2 teaspoons powdered Splenda

In a large mixing bowl, prepare the Jell-O as directed on the box.

Refrigerate until almost set but still a little soft, about 1 hour 15 minutes.

Beat the gelatin until creamy.

While continuing to beat with a mixer, add the cream cheese and sour cream. and mix thoroughly.

In another bowl, whip together whipping cream and Splenda until peaks form. Gently fold the whipped cream into the gelatin mixture, leaving it with a marbled look—don't keep stirring until it becomes uniform in color.

Spoon into dessert dishes and chill for at least 2 hours.

NANCY'S FANCY CHOCOLATE MERINGUE COOKIES

For Steps One, Two, and Three; **3 cookies = 5x5 carb**
Makes approximately 30 cookies

> 5 egg whites
>
> 1/4 teaspoon vinegar
>
> 1 1/2 teaspoons vanilla extract
>
> 1/2 cup granulated Splenda
>
> 1/4 cup Splenda "Sugar Blend for Baking"
>
> 1/4 cup unsweetened cocoa powder
>
> 1/4 cup ground pecans (optional)

Preheat the oven to 250°F. Line several cookie sheets with aluminum foil.

Whip egg whites until frothy. Add the vinegar and vanilla extract. Slowly add both kinds of Splenda. Beat until stiff.

Gently fold in the cocoa powder. Fold in the pecans, if using.

Using a tablespoon, spoon the mixture 1 inch apart, onto the prepared cookie sheets,

Bake for 2 hours.

Let cool and then peel gently from the foil.

Store in an airtight container.

Appendix: Fat Loss Expectations on Steps One and Two

WOMEN

Find your height and start-weight in the left hand columns to identify the number of "fat" pounds that you are expected to lose during the upcoming eight weeks on Steps One or Two. Remember, you will look like you have lost twice as much weight.

4'10" 90–130 lbs. = 3–5 lbs. fat loss
      130–170 = 6–13 lbs. fat loss
      170–210 = 14–21 lbs. fat loss
      210–250 = 22–29 lbs. fat loss

5'0" 100–140 lbs. = 3–5 lbs. fat loss
      140–180 lbs. = 6–13 lbs. fat loss
      180–220 lbs. = 14–21 lbs. fat loss
      220–260 lbs. = 22–29 lbs. fat loss

4'11" 95–135 lbs. = 3–5 lbs. fat loss
      135–175 lbs. = 6–13 lbs. fat loss
      175–215 lbs. = 14–21 lbs. fat loss
      215–255 lbs. = 22–29 lbs. fat los

5'1" 105–145 lbs. = 3–5 lbs. fat loss
      145–185 lbs. = 6–13 lbs. fat loss
      185–225 lbs. = 14–21 lbs. fat loss
      225–265 lbs. = 22–29 lbs. fat loss

5'2"   110–150 lbs. = 3–5 lbs. fat loss
        150–190 lbs. = 6–13 lbs. fat loss
        190–230 lbs. = 14–21 lbs. fat loss
        230–270 lbs. = 22–29 lbs. fat loss

5'3"   115–155 lbs. = 3–5 lbs. fat loss
        155–195 lbs. = 6–13 lbs. fat loss
        195–235 lbs. = 14–21 lbs. fat loss
        235–275 lbs. = 22–29 lbs. fat loss

5'4"   120–160 lbs. = 3–5 lbs. fat loss
        160–200 lbs. = 6–13 lbs. fat loss
        200–240 lbs. = 14–21 lbs. fat loss
        240–280 lbs. = 22–29 lbs. fat loss

5'5"   125–165 lbs. = 3–5 lbs. fat loss
        165–205 lbs. = 6–13 lbs. fat loss
        205–245 lbs. = 14–21 lbs. fat loss
        245–285 lbs. = 22–29 lbs. fat loss

5'6"   130–170 lbs. = 3–5 lbs. fat loss
        170–210 lbs. = 6–13 lbs. fat loss
        210–250 lbs. = 14–21 lbs. fat loss
        250–290 lbs. = 22–29 lbs. fat loss

5'7"   135–175 lbs. = 3–5 lbs. fat loss
        175–215 lbs. = 6–13 lbs. fat loss
        215–255 lbs. = 14–21 lbs. fat loss
        255–295 lbs. = 22–29 lbs. fat loss

5'8"   140–180 lbs. = 3–5 lbs. fat loss
        180–220 lbs. = 6–13 lbs. fat loss
        220–260 lbs. = 14–21 lbs. fat loss
        260–300 lbs. = 22–29 lbs. fat loss

5'9"   145–185 lbs. = 3–5 lbs. fat loss
        185–225 lbs. = 6–13 lbs. fat loss
        225–265 lbs. = 14–21 lbs. fat loss
        265–305 lbs. = 22–29 lbs. fat loss

5'10"   150–190 lbs. = 3–5 lbs. fat loss
        190–230 lbs. = 6–13 lbs. fat loss
        230–270 lbs. = 14–21 lbs. fat loss
        270–310 lbs. = 22–29 lbs. fat loss

5'11"   155–195 lbs. = 3–5 lbs. fat loss
        195–235 lbs. = 6–13 lbs. fat loss
        235–275 lbs. = 14–21 lbs. fat loss
        275–315 lbs. = 22–29 lbs. fat loss

6'0"   160–200 lbs. = 3–5 lbs. fat loss
        200–240 lbs. = 6–13 lbs. fat loss
        240–280 lbs. = 14–21 lbs. fat loss
        280–320 lbs. = 22–29 lbs. fat loss

MEN

Find your height and start-weight in the left hand columns to identify the number of "fat" pounds that you are expected to lose during the upcoming eight weeks on Steps One or Two. Remember, you will look like you have lost twice as much weight.

5'0"	106–146 lbs. = 3–5 lbs. fat loss		5'5"	136–176 lbs. = 3–5 lbs. fat loss	
	146–186 lbs. = 6–13 lbs. fat loss			176–216 lbs. = 6–13 lbs. fat loss	
	186–226 lbs. = 14–21 lbs. fat loss			216–256 lbs. = 14–21 lbs. fat loss	
	226–266 lbs. = 22–29 lbs. fat loss			256–296 lbs. = 22–29 lbs. fat loss	
5'1"	112–152 lbs. = 3–5 lbs. fat loss		5'6"	142–182 lbs. = 3–5 lbs. fat loss	
	152–192 lbs. = 6–13 lbs. fat loss			182–222 lbs. = 6–13 lbs. fat loss	
	192–232 lbs. = 14–21 lbs. fat loss			222–262 lbs. = 14–21 lbs. fat loss	
	232–272 lbs. = 22–29 lbs. fat loss			262–302 lbs. = 22–29 lbs. fat loss	
5'2"	118–158 lbs. = 3–5 lbs. fat loss		5'7"	148–188 lbs. = 3–5 lbs. fat loss	
	158–198 lbs. = 6–13 lbs. fat loss			188–228 lbs. = 6–13 lbs. fat loss	
	198–238 lbs. = 14–21 lbs. fat loss			228–268 lbs. = 14–21 lbs. fat loss	
	238–278 lbs. = 22–29 lbs. fat loss			268–308 lbs. = 22–29 lbs. fat loss	
5'3"	124–164 lbs. = 3–5 lbs. fat loss		5'8"	154–194 lbs. = 3–5 lbs. fat loss	
	164–204 lbs. = 6–13 lbs. fat loss			194–234 lbs. = 6–13 lbs. fat loss	
	204–244 lbs. = 14–21 lbs. fat loss			234–274 lbs. = 14–21 lbs. fat loss	
	244–284 lbs. = 22–29 lbs. fat loss			274–314 lbs. = 22–29 lbs. fat loss	
5'4"	130–170 lbs. = 3–5 lbs. fat loss		5'9"	160–200 lbs. = 3–5 lbs. fat loss	
	170–210 lbs. = 6–13 lbs. fat loss			200–240 lbs. = 6–13 lbs. fat loss	
	210–250 lbs. = 14–21 lbs. fat loss			240–280 lbs. = 14–21 lbs. fat loss	
	250–290 lbs. = 22–29 lbs. fat loss			280–320 lbs. = 22–29 lbs. fat loss	

5'10"   166–206 lbs. = 3–5 lbs. fat loss
206–246 lbs. = 6–13 lbs. fat loss
246–286 lbs. = 14–21 lbs. fat loss
286–326 lbs. = 22–29 lbs. fat loss

5'11"   172–212 lbs. = 3–5 lbs. fat loss
212–252 lbs. = 6–13 lbs. fat loss
252–292 lbs. = 14–21 lbs. fat loss
292–332 lbs. = 22–29 lbs. fat loss

6'0"   178–218 lbs. = 3–5 lbs. fat loss
218–258 lbs. = 6–13 lbs. fat loss
258–298 lbs. = 14–21 lbs. fat loss
298–338 lbs. = 22–29 lbs. fat loss

6'1"   184–224 lbs. = 3–5 lbs. fat loss
224-264 lbs. = 6–13 lbs. fat loss
264–304 lbs. = 14–21 lbs. fat loss
304–344 lbs. = 22–29 lbs. fat loss

6'2"   190–230 lbs. = 3–5 lbs. fat loss
230–270 lbs. = 6–13 lbs. fat loss
270–310 = 14–21 lbs. fat loss
210–350 lbs. = 22–29 lbs. fat loss

6'3"   196–236 lbs. = 3–5 lbs. fat loss
236–276 lbs. = 6–13 lbs. fat loss
276–316 lbs. = 14–21 lbs. fat loss
316–356 lbs. = 22–29 lbs. fat loss

6'4"   202–242 lbs. = 3–5 lbs. fat loss
242–282 lbs.-= 6–13 lbs. fat loss
282–322 lbs. = 14–21 lbs. fat loss
322–363 lbs. = 22=29 lbs. fat loss

6'5"   208–248 lbs. = 3–5 lbs. fat loss
248–288 lbs. = 6–13 lbs. fat loss
288–328 lbs. = 14–21 lbs. fat loss
328–368 lbs. = 22=29 lbs. fat loss

6'6"   214–254 lbs. = 3–5 lbs. fat loss
254–294 lbs. = 6–13 lbs. fat loss
294–334 lbs. = 14–21 lbs. fat loss
334–374 lbs. = 22–29 lbs. fat loss

Glossary

Anxiety, Panic Disorder: Many patients with Metabolism B report feelings of anxiety and nervousness that come and go. Some describe anxiety to the point of panic attacks that can cause shortness of breath, pounding or rapid heartbeat, cold sweats, dizziness, fainting, and shakiness. Although panic attacks exist for many reasons, there is definitely a relationship between panic attacks and blood sugar fluctuations. Treatment for blood sugar panic attacks would require stabilizing the blood sugar.

Attention Deficit Disorder or Attention-Deficit/Hyperactivity Disorder: ADD/ADHD is a neurobehavioral disorder affecting between 3 and 5 percent of children under the age of nineteen. Although it typically presents itself during childhood, it can last into adulthood. This disorder is usually treated by a combination of medications, behavior and lifestyle modifications, and counseling. Interestingly, many of the symptoms of ADD/ADHD are also the symptoms of progressing Metabolism B. It seems prudent to check the fasting blood glucose of children diagnosed with ADD/ADHD to see if changes in diet might help.

Blood Glucose: Also known as blood sugar, blood glucose is the body's fuel. The amount of glucose in the blood varies throughout the day and is hormonally regulated by the pancreas. Normal blood sugar is 65–140 mg/dL (3.6–7.8 mmol/L). Blood glucose can be stored in the muscles and liver as glycogen and excesses are stored as fat. Rises in blood glucose trigger the release of insulin. Drops in blood glucose trigger the release of glucagon.

Carbohydrate: A major nutrient found in many foods such as fruit, bread, legumes, milk, potatoes, rice, and pasta as well as sweets, desserts, and chips, carbohydrate converts 100 percent into blood glucose and is the body's preferred fuel source.

Chronic Fatigue: Also known as chronic fatigue syndrome, this type of exhaustion is an all-encompassing, draining fatigue. The person wakes up tired and remains drained throughout much of the day, making everyday life a real effort. People use the terms "washed out" or "totally drained" to describe this exhaustion. If Metabolism B is playing a part in chronic fatigue syndrome, then the hormonal balance that the Miracle provides will help alleviate this problem.

Depression (Mild): Depression is a physical medical condition involving an imbalance of brain chemicals. It is not diagnosed by a blood test but by the symptoms that the patient relates to the physician or therapist.

When a person's glucose level has sharp peaks and valleys, it causes many of the same symptoms that chemical depression causes. Because the symptoms sound so similar, the depression related to blood sugar imbalance is often misdiagnosed as chemical depression and is incorrectly treated with antidepressant medications. These patients often report little or no improvement even after the physician has changed the type or dose of antidepressant. Unfortunately, it is not commonly accepted that blood sugar imbalance can mimic the symptoms of brain chemical imbalance. It is probably prudent to check a patient's blood glucose level as part of a medical evaluation for depression. If fasting blood glucose exceeds 90 mg/dL (5 mmol/L), the Metabolism Miracle should be used (perhaps in tandem with medication for depression).

Diabetes

Prediabetes: Also known as borderline diabetes, prediabetes is a reversible condition. The diagnosis, made when fasting blood glucose is 100–125 mg/dL (5.6–6.9 mmol/L), is often considered a red flag that the patient is on the road to type 2 diabetes. With proper diet, exercise, and stress reduction, a diagnosis of type 2 diabetes may be prevented or forestalled. In an effort to be proactive, the Metabolism Miracle sets the red flag of prediabetes at 90–125 mg/dL (5–6.9 mmol/L).

Type 2 Diabetes: Type 2 diabetes, also known as adult onset diabetes, is the most common form of diabetes and is caused by either the pancreas not producing enough insulin and/or the insulin no longer fitting cells effectively (insulin resistance). Insulin is necessary for the body to use glucose for energy. It is the "key" that opens the cells so that they can accept the glucose from the bloodstream. If the pancreas does not produce enough insulin, or if the insulin can't open the cells appropriately, glucose has nowhere to go and subsequently builds up in the bloodstream. Type 2 diabetes is diagnosed with two fasting blood glucose tests over 125 mg/dL (6.9 mmol/L). Recurrent elevations of blood sugar can, over time, damage blood vessels and nerves, leading to irreversible complications involving the eyes, nerves, kidneys, blood vessels, and circulation.

Type 1 Diabetes: This is an autoimmune disease that results in the permanent destruction of insulin-producing beta cells in the pancreas. Its exact cause is unknown, but there appears to be a genetic link that may be precipitated by a virus or environmental trigger. Previously known as juvenile diabetes, its onset is usually abrupt. It is often diagnosed in children and young adults, but it can occur at any age. It results in the absence of insulin, and people with type 1 diabetes currently require insulin administration for life.

Gestational Diabetes (GDM): GDM occurs in a pregnant woman who has never had diabetes but develops high blood glucose during the pregnancy because normal placental hormones block the action of the mother's insulin. The pancreas fails to produce adequate insulin to bring the mother's blood glucose into normal range during the pregnancy. The treatment for GDM is diet modification, exercise as directed, and, in some cases, insulin injection. Most glucose levels normalize very soon after delivery. Babies born to mothers with untreated gestational diabetes often weigh 9 pounds or more.

Gestational diabetes is routinely screened between weeks 24 and 28 of the pregnancy. Approximately 6 percent of pregnant women develop GDM. Women with a history of GDM have a greater chance of a recurrence during future pregnancies and a greater chance of developing type 2 diabetes in the future.

Fasting Blood Glucose: Fasting blood glucose is determined by a lab test drawn first thing in the morning after at least eight hours without food or calorie-containing beverages. This test can be used to determine blood glucose conditions including prediabetes or type 2 diabetes. The American Diabetes Association normal fasting blood glucose level = 65–99 mg/dL (3.6–5.5 mmol/L). Prediabetes = 100–125 mg/dL (5.6–6.9 mmol/L) (inclusive). Diabetes = *greater than or equal to* 126 mg/dL (7 mmol/L). The diagnosis of diabetes should be confirmed with a second fasting blood glucose result *greater than or equal to* 126 mg/dL.

Fat Cells: The number of fat cells you will carry throughout life is determined in utero and can again increase at the beginning of puberty. When an adult gains weight, it is the size and not the number of fat cells that increases.

Fibromyalgia: This constellation of symptoms includes fatigue, muscle pain, and stiffness. It also often includes constipation, headaches, decreased short-term memory, decreased ability to focus thoughts, menstrual cramping, numbness, tingling, dizziness, and skin sensitivity. Many of these symptoms overlap with the symptoms of insulin resistance, metabolic syndrome, prediabetes, hypoglycemia, and type 2 diabetes. These symptoms markedly improve for many people with Metabolism B when they follow the Miracle program.

GERD (Gastric Reflux Disease): GERD often occurs in people who have a hiatal hernia. Similar to the way that increased midline fat can affect sleep apnea, the extra fat stores around the middle can press on the stomach and cause stomach acid to backflow into the esophagus. Weight loss around the middle drastically decreases GERD's symptoms.

Glucagon: A pancreatic hormone that signals the liver to release glycogen stores and effectively stops blood glucose from dropping lower than the normal range.

Glycemic Index: Also referred to as GI, this is an index that ranks carbohydrates based on the rate at which they convert to blood glucose. The glycemic index has a scale of 0–100, with higher values given to foods that cause the most rapid rise in blood sugar. Pure glucose is the reference point and it is given a GI of 100. For simple comparison, the foods are ranked according to their same size in weight, 50 grams. It is important to note, however, that the GI is not based on typical portion size of the food (see next entry).

Glycemic Load: GL ranks the glycemic index of foods according to the "typical" portion size of that particular food.

Glycogen: Glycogen is glucose that is formed and stored in muscle cells and in the liver. Glycogen is released from the muscles when a person exercises and is released from the liver if a person skips or delays a meal or during the sleep hours. When glycogen is released, it causes blood glucose to rise into the normal range.

Hunger: Hunger is a natural physical phenomenon. It is an unpleasant feeling experienced when one's blood sugar level begins to drop four to five hours after a meal and when the glycogen level of the liver drops below a certain threshold. The feeling associated with hunger gives us the signal to eat.

Hypertension (High Blood Pressure): Blood pressure consists of two readings: The upper reading is known as systolic and is the pressure created when your heart beats. It is considered high if it exceeds 140 mmHg. The lower reading, diastolic, is a measure of the pressure inside your blood vessels when the heart is at rest. It is considered elevated if it exceeds 90mmHg. The current recommended blood pressure goal is less than 130/80 mmHg.

Hypertension is directly related to excess weight. For those with untreated Metabolism B, continual, gradual weight gain is a matter of fact. As weight increases, so, too, does blood pressure. The permanent weight loss effected by the Metabolism Miracle will quickly help to decrease blood pressure.

Hypoglycemia: There are two types of hypoglycemia. One is caused by the excess insulin of Metabolism B while the other is drug induced from excess glucose lowering medication for diabetes. This temporary state of low blood sugar may come with symptoms of shaking, light-headedness, confusion, irritability, hunger, carb cravings, cold sweats, and headache. Eating carbohydrate food immediately relieves the symptoms.

Hypoglycemia is generally classified when blood sugar dips below 70 mg/dL (3.9 mmol/L) or lower. With unchecked Metabolism B, the symptoms can occur one and a half to three hours after a meal, when the overactive pancreas pumps out excess insulin. Symptoms of hypoglycemia due to excess insulin release is a precursor to prediabetes and ultimately type 2 diabetes. A person with normal metabolism should not experience hypoglycemia. (For treatment of hypoglycemia, see chapter 12, page 196).

Hypothyroidism: Thyroid hormones determine the speed of metabolism. When the thyroid gland can't produce enough hormone, the metabolic rate slows. Symptoms include fatigue, weakness, weight gain, or difficulty losing weight. Dry skin, constipation, muscle cramps, cold intolerance, depression, irritability, memory loss, abnormal menstrual cycles, and depressed libido can also be related to hypothyroidism. Many of the symptoms for insulin resistance, metabolic syndrome, hypoglycemia, prediabetes, and type 2 diabetes are the same. Simple blood tests are used to determine if thyroid levels are adequate and if blood sugar is in target range. Only with blood tests can one determine hypothyroidism or blood glucose abnormalities.

Injectable Insulin: Used as a medical treatment for diabetes, injectable insulin is manufactured in the laboratory using recombinant DNA.

Insulin: The hormone insulin, produced by the pancreas, helps *lower* blood glucose. Insulin acts like a key and opens the doorways into your fat and muscle cells allowing excess glucose in your blood to move into the opened fat and muscle cells. This movement brings blood glucose back into the normal range. It also enables the glucose to be used for energy (muscle cells) or stored as fat (fat cells). Insulin is a storage hormone.

Insulin Resistance: Insulin resistance occurs when the normal amount of insulin secreted by the pancreas is not able to work effectively. When insulin does not "fit" the cell's receptors appropriately, it cannot work effectively. Eventually, the pancreas cannot keep up with the body's need for insulin, and excess glucose builds up in the bloodstream. Ironically, many people with insulin resistance have high levels of blood glucose and high levels of insulin circulating in their blood at the same time.

Liver: The liver contains a stockpile of blood sugar in the form of glycogen. Whenever you choose to skip or delay a meal and every night while you are asleep, it is your liver's release of glycogen that keeps you alive. Through the liver's intervention, the human body has the ability to "self-feed."

Metabolic Syndrome: This group of conditions increases your risk for diabetes, heart disease, and stroke. Symptoms include increased blood pressure, elevated insulin levels, excess body fat around the waist, elevated LDL cholesterol, elevated triglycerides, decreased HDL cholesterol, prediabetes, and type 2 diabetes. A major root cause of metabolic syndrome is insulin resistance.

Midline Fat Deposits: One of the hallmarks of this genetic predisposition to Metabolism B is a roll of fat around the middle. Some people also note increased "back fat." This hallmark fat deposit around the middle even occurs in otherwise thin patients.

Net Carbohydrate: The amount of carbohydrate that will eventually convert to blood glucose. Net carbohydrate is *included* in the total carbohydrate grams on a food label. Use the following formula to determine net carbs:

Total carbohydrate grams - dietary fiber grams = net carbohydrate grams
    Never subtract "sugar alcohol" from total carbohydrate to find a net carb, as a portion of sugar alcohol grams will convert to blood glucose.

Normal Blood Glucose Range: A person with normal carbohydrate metabolism will have blood glucose between 65 and 140 mg/dL (3.6 and 7.8 mmol/L) regardless of what he or she chooses to eat or not eat. In terms of normal blood glucose metabolism, a person can choose to fast for two days or eat a half pound of pasta with a loaf of garlic bread, and in either case, his or her blood glucose will remain in the 65–140 mg/dL range. Blood glucose is hormonally regulated by the pancreas with the help of the hormones insulin and glucagon.

Osteoarthritis: OA, a low-grade inflammation and decreased lubricating fluid in the joints, causes abnormal wearing of the protective cartilage that covers the joints. As the protection of the joints decreases, simple activities such as walking and standing become painful. Activity gradually decreases, which can compromise the functioning of muscles and ligaments. Increased body weight caused by metabolic syndrome causes osteoarthritis to be more painful and advance faster.

Osteopenia: Osteopenia occurs when bone density dips below normal. Regular exercise along with calcium and vitamin D supplementation help to alleviate the problem. If left untreated, osteopenia can lead to osteoporosis.

Osteoporosis: In this disease, bone mineral density is so compromised that an increased risk of bone fracture results. Hypothyroidism and type 2 diabetes contribute to the condition. Regular exercise, along with calcium and vitamin D supplementation, helps to prevent the condition.

Pancreas: The dual function gland/organ responsible for producing hormones that regulate blood sugar (insulin and glucagon) and digestive enzymes. Insulin and glucagon keep blood glucose in the normal range of 65–140 mg/dL (3.6–7.8 mmol/L).

Polycystic Ovarian Syndrome (PCOS): This endocrine disorder affects more than 10 percent of all women. Possibly caused by insulin resistance and the genes related to type 2 diabetes, its symptoms include irregular, few, or absent menstrual periods; depression; acne, oily skin, or dark patches of skin; infertility; hirsutism (excessive or increased body hair affecting face, chest, legs); and insulin resistance.

Sleep Apnea: In this sleep disorder, long pauses in breathing during sleep cause people to miss a number of breaths throughout the night. Lifestyle changes, such as weight loss, help arrest the loud snoring, restless sleep, and daytime sleepiness that go along with sleep apnea. Untreated Metabolism B accumulates fat around the middle, which puts pressure on the diaphragm during sleep. The Metabolism Miracle's fat burning steps decrease midline fat and help decrease pressure on the diaphragm, thereby helping to alleviate sleep apnea.

Sleep Disturbance: Two different sleep disturbances occur with uncontrolled Metabolism B. One is the inability of the brain to relax and allow the person to fall asleep, even when the body is legitimately tired. The other disturbance occurs when a person falls asleep easily, awakens in the middle of the night, and cannot return to sleep. Both sleep disturbances seem to be caused by peaks and valleys of blood sugar during the night.

Acknowledgments

Michael Scott Simon, Esq.: My heartfelt thanks for your involvement in every step of the way as *The Metabolism Miracle* progressed from my dream to a reality. Your endless energy, enthusiasm, perfectionism, tenacity, and support helped me from the first day of this project. I can never thank you enough, TB.

Andrea Somberg: My agent at the Harvey Klinger agency. Thank you for seeing the promise in the manuscript and for working to get it into the best hands.

Matthew Lore: My original publisher and editor. Your energy, intelligence, professionalism, and creativity have been greatly appreciated throughout the initial phase of this process. Thank you for taking on my life's work, recognizing the importance of "the Miracle," being open-minded through the entire process, and patiently teaching me the ropes.

Wendy Francis: Senior Editor. Thank you for taking over *The Metabolism Miracle* in the middle of the game. You have been positive, calm, collected, and professional. Thanks for all you did to make "The Miracle" a reality. Kudos to you!

Allison Cleary: My editor/writer and friend. Thank you so very much for all you put into the editing of *The Metabolism Miracle*. You are a phenomenal writer and editor with a God-given talent for making concepts come to life. You were an absolute pleasure to work with, always professional, always open, ever-sharing, a consummate professional. I look forward to working with you again in future endeavors!!!!!!!!!!!!!!!!!!

Wendie Carr and Perseus Publicity Department. Thank you for the interest, professionalism, and help you channeled into publicizing the Miracle.

Cisca Schreefel, senior project editor, and Iris Bass, copy editor. Thank you for the meticulous job you did with this project. Your creativity, knowledge, and perfectionism is greatly appreciated.

Lindsey Triebel, marketing manager, and the marketing department at Da Capo Lifelong Books. Thanks for the energy, enthusiasm, and professionalism you invested in the marketing of the Miracle.

Phil Kresefski: My husband and childhood sweetheart. You've been by my side since we were children. Thank you for standing beside me in all of life's adventures. You always encourage me to be creative, trust in myself, stay positive, and work toward my dreams. Thank you for your patience and help during the countless hours involved in this process.

Diana Kresefski: My daughter and best friend. You have been a consistent source of strength, encouragement, laughs, and reality checks. You are wise beyond your years and are sure to go far in your life. Thank you for working beside me every day and keeping the Nutrition Center of Morristown (NCOM) running smoothly. I am so very proud of you.

Phillip Kresefski: My son, my heart. Thank you for your support and love. You are already an accomplished student-athlete, and a wonderful, caring son. I am so very proud of you.

Ann and Bill Haduch: My parents. Your life's example motivated me to persevere, push the limits, strive for success, and above all . . .keep a positive attitude. Because of your influence, I appreciate the beauty that life has to offer.

Raymond Kresefski, Sr.: My father-in-law, the finest human being I've ever met: strong, selfless, caring, unconditionally loving. I am thankful to have had you in my life. Rest in peace.

Edward Shebol: God bless you, Grandpa. Thank you for always being there with your strength, intelligence, humor, and prayers.

(JI, DG, DF), (MN, RC, CC, TC, GS, SS): Thank you for fueling my fire to move on. Without your influence, I would never have chosen the path that led to this book.

Carmella Kresefski: Thank you for the countless hours you spent with me during the writing of this book.

My wonderful patients from the NCOM: A special thank-you to all of my patients (many of whom I count among my friends) whom I've worked with at the Nutrition Center of Morristown. Your insights, trials/tribulations, successes, and your lives are intertwined on every page of *The Metabolism Miracle*. Thank you for everything you have taught me along the way. I wish all of you all of the best.

About the Author

Diane Kress, RD CDE, is a registered dietitian and certified diabetes educator with more than twenty-five years' experience in medical nutrition therapy. She is well known in the New York–New Jersey–Connecticut tristate area as a leading authority on innovative diet counseling. After years of practicing as a traditional nutritionist, she researched and developed the proprietary program presented in this book, specifically for those patients who could not succeed with traditional diets. *The Metabolism Miracle* has already provided over three thousand of her private practice patients with remarkable results involving permanent weight loss and decreased medications with improved blood sugar, blood pressure, cholesterol, and overall well-being.

Diane Kress's specialty areas include dietary treatment of morbid obesity, weight reduction, diabetes management and prevention, metabolic syndrome, and cardiac care nutrition. She has worked in the clinical settings of hospitals, has consulted for school systems, and currently owns and directs her own private practice, the Nutrition Center of Morristown, in Morristown, New Jersey.

Kress is a member of the American Dietetic Association, American Association of Diabetes Educators, and American Diabetes Association and has been affiliated with the Garden State Association of Diabetes Educators. She has authored articles for newspapers and is a well-known speaker at medical programs throughout New Jersey. She lives in New Jersey with her husband and two children.

Index

Numbers in bold indicate boxed text.